Steroid Hormone Action and Cancer

CURRENT TOPICS IN MOLECULAR ENDOCRINOLOGY

Series Editors: Bert W. O'Malley and Anthony R. Means
Department of Cell Biology
Baylor College of Medicine
Houston, Texas

Volume 1: *Hormone Binding and Target Cell Activation in the Testis*
Edited by Maria L. Dufau and Anthony R. Means

Volume 2: *Hormonal Regulation of Spermatogenesis*
Edited by Frank S. French, Vidar Hansson, E. Martin Ritzen, and Shihadeh N. Nayfeh

Volume 3: *Hypothalamus and Endocrine Functions*
Edited by Fernand Labrie, Joseph Meites, and Georges Pelletier

Volume 4: *Steroid Hormone Action and Cancer*
Edited by K.M.J. Menon and Jerry R. Reel

Steroid Hormone Action and Cancer

Edited by

K. M. J. Menon
University of Michigan Medical School
Ann Arbor, Michigan

and

Jerry R. Reel
Parke Davis Research Laboratories
Ann Arbor, Michigan

PLENUM PRESS · NEW YORK AND LONDON

Library of Congress Cataloging in Publication Data

Main entry under title:

Steroid hormone action and cancer.

(Current topics in molecular endocrinology; v. 4)
Based on the proceedings of a conference held at the University of Michigan, Ann Arbor, Oct. 27-29, 1975, and sponsored by the Dept. of Postgraduate Medicine and Health Professions Education.
Includes index.
1. Cancer–Chemotherapy–Congresses. 2. Steroid hormones–Therapeutic use–Congresses. 3. Hormone receptors–Congresses. 4. Hormone antagonists–Congresses. I. Menon, Karumathil Matathil Jayaram. II. Reel, J. R. III. Michigan, University. Dept. of Postgraduate Medicine and Health Professions Education. [DNLM: 1. Steroids–Therapeutic use–Congresses. 2. Steroids–Pharmacodynamics–Congresses. 3. Neoplasms–Drug therapy–Congresses. QZ267 S839 1975]
RC271.H55S73 616.9'94'061 76-25873

ISBN-13: 978-1-4684-2603-8 e-ISBN-13: 978-1-4684-2601-4
DOI: 10.1007/978-1-4684-2601-4

Proceedings of a symposium on Steroid Hormone Action and Cancer held at the University of Michigan, Ann Arbor, Michigan, October 27-29, 1975

Softcover reprint of the hardcover 1st edition 1976

A Division of Plenum Publishing Corporation
227 West 17th Street, New York, N.Y. 10011

Preface

This volume is an outgrowth of a symposium held at the University of Michigan, Ann Arbor, Michigan, October 27-29, 1975. This symposium was organized to bring together basic scientists and clinicians for the purpose of exchanging new ideas and the latest information in the area of Steroid Hormone Action and Cancer. The design of the symposium included both formal plenary sessions and informal roundtable discussion groups, the chapters of this volume being drawn primarily from these proceedings.

During the last quarter of a century considerable progress has been made toward understanding the molecular mechanisms involved in steroid hormone action. It now appears that the mechansim of action of the four major classes of steroid hormones is qualitatively similar. Research during the past decade has demonstrated steroid hormone receptors in a variety of normal and neoplastic tissues. Receptor-containing neoplasms have been shown to be hormone-dependent and undergo regression when treated with hormone antagonists. Natural and synthetic steroids also have been employed for many years to successfully treat various types of cancer, for example: estrogens, androgens and progestagens for breast cancer; estrogens and progestagens for prostatic carcinoma; progestagens for endometrial carcinoma; and corticoids for leukemias. All of these neoplasms have now been found to possess receptors for the steroids empirically used in their treatment. By analogy to the known relationship between estrogen receptors and the response of breast cancer to endocrine therapies, the latter observations suggest that steroid receptors may have prognostic value in deciding which neoplasms will respond to hormonal therapy.

The editors would like to thank all members of the Conference Committee for their efforts in organizing this symposium, and for serving as moderators of the roundtable discussions. We also are indebted to the Department of Postgraduate Medicine and Health Professions Education, University of Michigan, who sponsored this meeting and to the following pharmaceutical companies who provided financial support: Ayerst, Eli Lilly, Hoffman-LaRoche, McNeil, Ortho, Ciba, Geigy, Searle, Upjohn and Wyeth.

The excellent cooperation and efforts of Ms. Phyllis M. Straw and Mr. Stephen Dyer and other members of the staff of Plenum Press are gratefully acknowledged. Finally, we wish to thank Mrs. Cynthia Giraud for her time, effort and excellent cooperation in typing the manuscripts.

Contents

1. Steroid-Induced, Steroid-Producing and Steroid-Responsive Tumors 1
Roy Hertz

2. The Etiology of Breast Cancer 15
Marvin A. Rich, Philip Furmanski, Charles M. McGrath, Justin McCormick, Jose Russo and Herbert Soule

3. Selecting Endocrine Therapy in Breast Cancer 28
W.L. McGuire, K.B. Horwitz and M. De La Garza

4. The Metabolism of Steroid Hormones in Breast Cancer: A Reappraisal 36
S.C. Brooks

5. Fractionation of Diverse Steroid-Binding Proteins: Basic and Clinical Applications 51
Merry R. Sherman and Lorraine K. Miller

6. Mammalian Progesterone Receptors: Biosynthesis, Structure, and Nuclear Binding 68
L.E. Faber, J. Saffran, T.H. Chen and W.W. Leavitt

7. The Mode of Action of Progestagens on Endometrial Carcinoma 85
Jerry R. Reel

8. Are Oral Contraceptives and Diethylstilbestrol (DES) Involved in Sex-Linked Cancer? 95
Richard A. Edgren

9. Radioiodinated Estrogens and Antiestrogens as Potential Imaging Agents 107
R.E. Counsell, A. Buswink, N. Korn, M. Johnson, V. Ranade, and T. Yu

10. The Cellular Actions of Glucocorticoids in Relation to Human Neoplasms 114
E. Brad Thompson

11. Adrenal Steroids, Membranes and Neoplasia 133
Thomas D. Gelehrter

12. Active Forms and Biodynamics of the Androgen-Receptor in Various Target Tissues 139
Shutsung Liao, Stephen C. Hung, John L. Tymoczko and Tehming Liang

13. The Relevance of Studies on Androgen Action to Prostatic Cancer 152
W. Ian P. Mainwaring

14. Summary 172
K.M.J. Menon

Conference Committee 176

Index 177

STEROID-INDUCED, STEROID-PRODUCING, AND STEROID-RESPONSIVE TUMORS

Roy Hertz

Department of Pharmacology
The George Washington University Medical Center
Washington, D.C.

As an introduction to the chapters to follow, this report will aim to present certain hopefully provocative observations on the nature of steroid-related tumors in man and animals.

Steroids constitute a class of compounds which have as their common denominator their adherence to the cyclopentenophenanthrene structure (Fig 1). Although we conventionally categorize the hormonal steroids as either estrogens, progestins, corticoids or androgens, it is more realistic to consider that the steroids exhibit a continuous spectrum of biological effects. For example, the mineralocorticoid, deoxycorticosterone possesses about 5% of the progestational action of progesterone itself. Testosterone will in some species exert the type of uterotrophic action usually attributed to the estrogens (1). Several of the synthetic progestins have both androgenic and estrogenic potency (2). Thus the specificity of the characteristic biological effects of many steroids is relative rather than absolute and a considerable degree of overlap is frequently encountered.

In addition, certain classes of steroids may either synergize or neutralize the expected effects of other steroids. The well-known antagonism between estrogen and androgen has been long appreciated (3). A similar antagonism between estrogens and progesterone is readily demonstrated in such systems as the rabbit uterus (4) and the avian genital tract (5) (Fig 2). However, in lower dosage combinations a synergistic action between estrogen and progesterone is demonstrable (4,5). One of the potent synthetic progestins, namely cyproterone acetate, exhibits a marked anti-androgenic action as well (6). Progesterone has weak-anti-aldosterone action, but the

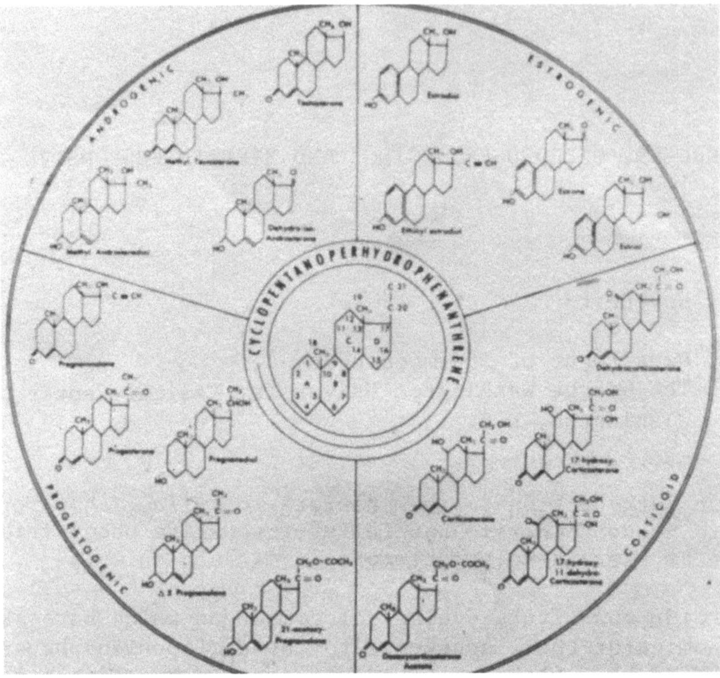

Fig 1. Spectrum of Steroid Hormones

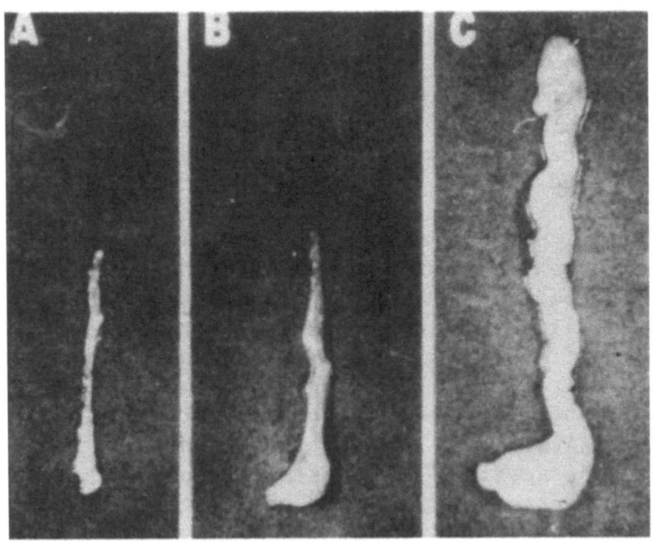

Fig 2. Chick Oviducts. A) Untreated; B) Estrogen and progesterone; and C) Estrogen alone.

synthetic spironolactones whose primary action is anti-aldosterone are weak progestins (7,8).

Hence, when one throws a steroid pebble into the vast metabolic pool, the resulting ripples may extend in varied physiological directions and we should not too rigidly characterize steroids as estrogens, progestins, corticoids or androgens.

It is now clearly established that both the qualitative and quantitative tissue response to steroid hormones varies with the genetic constitution of the subject. Dorfman demonstrated many years ago that the comb-growth response in various breeds of chicks will vary substantially (9). Thus, the White Leghorn will give a marked comb-growth response to a dose of androgen which yields no significant response in the Barred Rock (9) (Fig 3). Bardin et al (10,11) and Ohno and Lyon (12) indicate that the genetically determined insensitivity of such normally androgen-responsive tissues as the sub-maxillary gland, and the preputial gland of mice and rats with the testicular feminization syndrome lack essential receptor

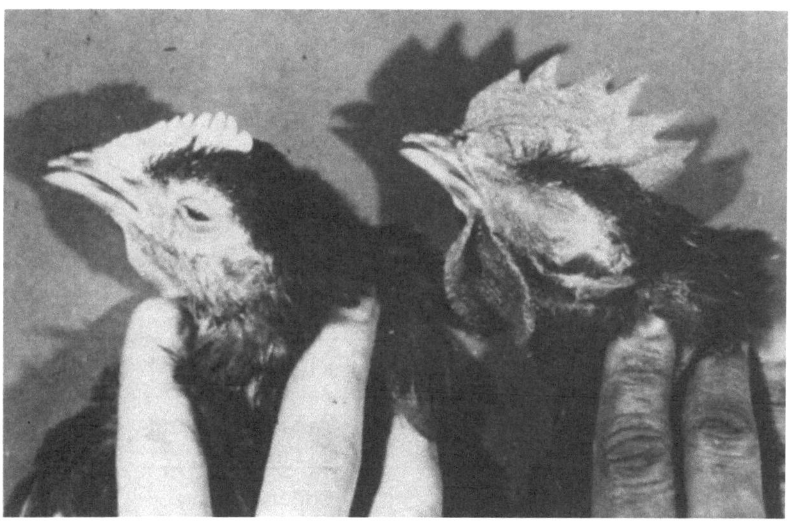

Fig 3. Androgenic Response in Chick Comb. Left - untreated control; Right - testosterone-treated.

sites for such response (13). There appears then to be emerging a stimulating study of the genetic aspects of endocrinology which may serve to elucidate further our growing knowledge of the cellular and of even the chromosomal basis for steroid action.

The problem of hormone-induced tumors bears directly on this issue of the genetic factors involved. More specifically, steroid-induced tumors in animals have provided data of great theoretical and practical importance. Table I lists both the species and organs in which a wide range of tumors has been produced, by estrogens. More recently certain progestins and estrogen-progestin combinations have also elicited ovarian tumors in mice and mammary tumors in Beagle dogs. The multiplicity of sites and species reflects a rather widely distributed susceptibility for such response. However, the exacting genetic requirements for such an effect have been an intrinsic part of the available data (14,15). Thus, high tumor strains are observed to be more susceptible to tumor induction by exogenous steroid than low tumor strains. The more recent knowledge of the role of hormonal binding sites in determining endocrine responsiveness to hormonal alteration in established breast cancer (16,17) and endometrial cancer (18) which will be reviewed in this volume has yet to be extended to the genetic aspect of the pathogenetic phase of these experimentally-induced tumors.

TABLE I

Estrogen-Induced Tumors

Species	Site
Mouse	Mammary Gland Cervix Testis Pituitary Bone Marrow Adrenal
Hamster	Kidney
Rat	Mammary Gland Pituitary
Rabbit	Endometrium
Dog	Ovary
Squirrel Monkey	Uterus
Human (Embryo)	Vagina Cervix

The data summarized in Table I also stress the critical role of dosage and duration of exposure to exogenous steroid in tumor induction. Actually, detailed dose-response data for this effect are surprisingly sparse. However, it would seem that most of the dosages employed over the years would substantially raise the steroid blood level above the endogenous level. Moreover, in most of the reported experiments the duration of exposure has equalled a significant portion of the life span of the species involved. Also, the earlier in life the hormone exposure has been initiated, the more readily have tumors been elicited (14).

An additional feature of the experimental experience has been the remarkable lack of specificity in the chemical structure required for estrogen-induced tumor formation (14). Thus both steroid and stilbene estrogens have proven comparably effective in equivalent estrogenic dosage for the respective species (Fig 5).

It is instructive to attempt to relate our experimental appreciation of the role of age, dosage, duration of exposure, and genetic determinants to the occurrence of vaginal or cervical adenocarcinoma and of adenosis of the daughters of women treated with synthetic non-steroidal estrogens during early pregnancy (19,20,21).

With respect to the genetic aspect, we must emphasize that the human population is of such extreme genetic heterogeneity that a low level of response is to be expected. Thus Lanier et al reviewed 819 cases of exposed females without identifying a single instance of carcinoma (22). Ulfelder (23) on the basis of prescription data of Heinonen (24) estimates that the attack rate among exposed offspring will be about 0.2%. This low level of response is what would be expected in a genetically unselected population. It may very well be that our genetic variability is our best protection against such exogenous influences. However the occurrence of some degree of vaginal adenosis in over 90% of those exposed and in all girls presenting with carcinoma suggests that this less ominous lesion requires much more commonly distributed genetic determinants than those essential for carcinoma induction. This view is supported by the observation that thus far no clinical or histological evidence of progression from adenosis to carcinoma has been observed (23).

As to dosage and duration of exposure, most cases have been associated with sustained medication throughout the prenatal period and with truly massive dosage. However, there are recorded a few cases following very brief exposure at dosages commonly employed in daily clinical practice (23). Although such data provide no basis for deriving a dose-response curve, the observations to date indicate a very critical period during organogenesis of the female genital tract for carcinoma induction. It would therefore seem desirable

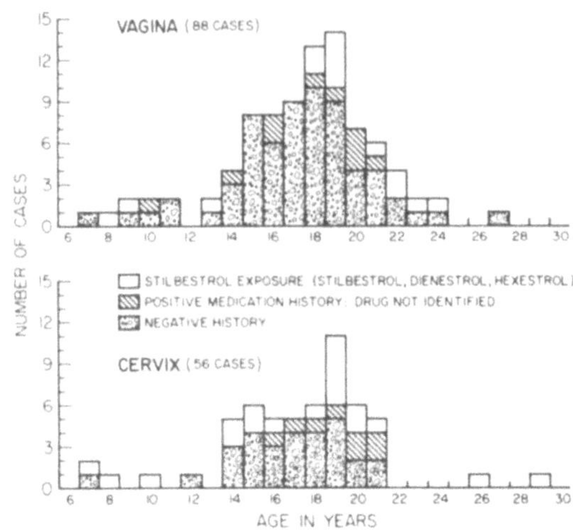

Fig 4. Age Distribution of Cases of Vaginal Adenocarcinoma (from Herbst et al, 1971).

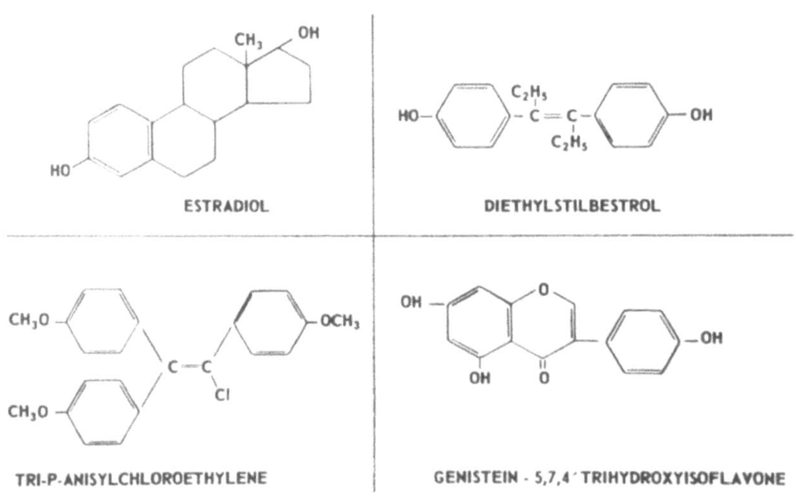

Fig 5. Variety of Structures of Estrogenic Compounds.

to consider this type of response to be a teratocarcinogenic effect rather than a classical carcinogenic effect.

Nevertheless, the interval between exposure and the clinical presentation of disease is highly characteristic for known human carcinogenic response. Fig 4 presents Dr. Herbst's data on the age distribution of the first cases reported. It is apparent that the latent period for the clinical response ranges from one to two decades (19). In comparison, Table II represents Dr. Heuper's tabulation of the characteristic latent period for known human carcinogens (25). The similarity is very striking.

TABLE II

Latent Period for Known Human Carcinogens*

Carcinogen	Site of Cancer	Range of Latency, yr.
X-rays	Skin	10-30
Radioactive paints	Bone	10-30
Radioactive ores	Lung	5-20
Thorium dioxide	Liver	10-25
Ultraviolet exposure	Skin	10-40
Aromatic amines	Bladder	2-20
Coal tar (shale oil)	Skin	10-25
Soot (chimney sweeps)	Scrotum	11-17

*From Heuper (25) (Table 1. Latent Period of Some Known Carcinogens in Man)

The clinical experience to date indicates that only the non-steroidal type of estrogen has been associated with these phenomena. However, our animal data indicate that the estrogenic response, unlike the other steroid-hormonal tissue responses may be induced by compounds of a wide variety of structures (Fig 5). Since diethylstilbestrol in the dosages utilized by the exposed pregnant women would cost only a fraction of the equivalent dosages of steroid preparations, a strong factor of selection in favor of this form of estrogen in the large dosages utilized would apply. It would seem unwise then to interpret the present clinical observations as necessarily indicating that a selective action of non-steroidal estrogens as opposed to steroidal estrogens actually exists for man as contrasted with experimental animals.

The relationship between endogenous or exogenous estrogens and endometrial cancer has been previously reviewed (26). More recently Cutler et al have reported six cases of endometrial cancer in young women chronically treated with stilbestrol for correction of the estrogen deficiency of Turner's syndrome (27). Here again the therapy was sustained for from 4 to 20 years, having been begun in the late teens or early twenties. A registry now includes 28 such cases. Most unusual is the very high frequency of an adenosquamous type of endometrial carcinoma in these women. This histological pattern is somewhat analogous to the squamous metaplasia produced in the rodent endometrium and in the cervical epithelium of the rhesus monkey by chronic estrogen exposure (28). In the rhesus monkey, this effect could be completely prevented by simultaneous administration of progesterone (29). Moreover, Reagan has noted an annual increment in the proportion of adenosquamous endometrial carcinomas in women from 3% to 30% of the cases seen over the past 35 years of experience in his laboratory (29).

However, it should be noted that patients with Turner's syndrome are mostly dysgenetic individuals, usually presenting an XO or mosaic karyotype. Whereas it is known that such dysgenetic patterns are associated with a relatively high frequency of neoplasms in the primitive gonadal anlagen of such patients, spontaneous occurrence of malignancy in the endometrium or in other Müllerian derivatives is recorded for only one aged patient with Turner's syndrome. Thus the effect observed by Cutler et al (27) is both quantitatively and qualitatively arresting.

Meanwhile, Smith and Hertman have provided a case-controlled retrospective study of the relative risk of endometrial cancer among 317 estrogen treated menopausal women as compared with the risk of other gynecological neoplasms among an equal number of aged-matched estrogen-treated controls (30). Their data indicate a five-fold increment in risk for endometrial cancer over the control level. The careful epidemiological design of this study lends some credence to the plethora of earlier statistically invalid studies purporting to demonstrate this relationship (31). It would be highly desirable to have much more comprehensive studies of this problem since it is advocated by many that all women over 40 should be placed on estrogen therapy for the remainder of their life-span.

An additional instance of steroid-related neoplasia in young women is the occurrence thus far of 20 cases of primary hepatic adenoma with an invariable association in all reported cases with the use of estrogen-progestin preparations (32). All but 3 of these cases are associated with a prior exposure of from 3 to 8 years, the remaining 3 cases ranging from one half to two years of exposure. Much remains to be learned about the epidemiological relationships involved in this phenomenon, but there is a striking similarity between these hepatic lesions in women and the focal nodular hyperplasia produced in rats by chronically-fed high dosage of mestranol, the most commonly used estrogen in the contraceptives utilized by these women.

Let us turn now from the hormone-induced tumors to a few instructive experiences with steroid-producing tumors.

It is noteworthy that steroidogenic tumors arise exclusively in organs which normally produce steroids - namely the ovary, testis, and adrenal. In contrast, tumors producing protein hormones such as adrenocorticotrophic hormone or chorionic gonadotropin arise not only in the pituitary or in the trophoblast but in a wide variety of tissues, thus constituting the new clearly delineated "ectopic" hormonal syndromes readily recognized in bronchogenic carcinomas, melanomas, gastro-intestinal tumors, and many other neoplastic lesions. The lack of as yet recognizable primarily steroidogenic ectopic tumors, suggests that the steroid-producing function represents a more highly specialized biosynthetic process than the presumably more primitive formation of protein hormones. This view is supported by the fact that the protein hormone, chorionic gonadotropin is produced in abundance as early in ontogenetic development as implantation or even before.

Among the steroid-producing tumors, those arising in the adrenal cortex have yielded to most extensive endocrinological and pharmacological manipulation. For example, the loss of negative feedback demonstrable by failure of suppression by exogenous corticoid in adrenal adenoma and in adrenal carcinoma as contrasted with adrenal hyperplasia connotes a remarkable alteration in the hypothalamic-pituitary relationship when neoplasia occurs. The pathogenetic import of such endocrinologic alteration merits further clinical as well as experimental analysis with modern methods of mensuration of the pituitary and hypothalamic factors involved.

More recently developed pharmacological agents for the metabolic and therapeutic manipulation of steroid-producing tumors of the adrenal cortex offer a special opportunity for such study. The direct interference with steroid biosynthesis in hormone-producing adrenal cancers by such compounds as metyrapone, amphenone, and aminoglutethimide have been clearly dissociated from any oncolytic action on these tumors (33,34,35). Clinically, no regressions of primary or metastic adrenal tumor were elicited by these agents, although the metabolic burden of the excessively produced steroids can be substantially reduced by these compounds.

In marked contrast the specific cytolytic action of o,p'-DDD on adrenal cortical cells not only reduces the metabolic effects of hyperadrenocorticism but also induces regression of tumor in about one third of the cases (36,37).

In the light of the respective and contrasting effects of these two differing types of agents, it becomes clear that the growth potential of the neoplastic as well as of the normal adrenocortical cell is readily separable from its steroidogenic function. This differentiation merits more extensive biochemical and cytological analysis than it has received to date.

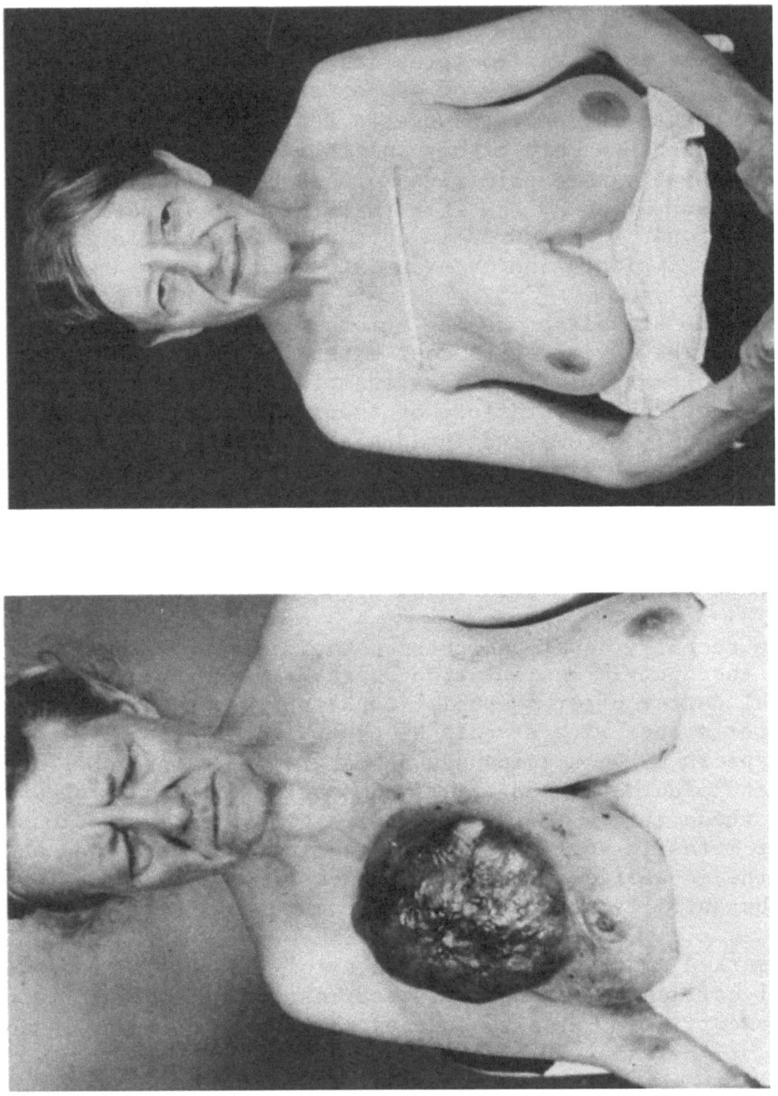

Fig 6. Histologically Proven, Previously Untreated Breast Cancer: Left - before therapy; Right - after stilbestrol therapy.

The last category of steroid-related tumors which we wish to discuss is that of the steroid-responsive tumors. In this instance we are speaking of the effects upon clinically established malignancy.

The most extensively studied lesion in this regard is that of cancer of the breast. The remarkable effects of ablative and additive hormonal manipulation of human breast cancer are covered by McGuire's chapter in this volume. However, by way of introduction to these studies on breast cancer, permit me to share with you a most remarkable clinical experience in this area in the case of this striking regression of a histologically proven and previously untreated breast cancer in an elderly women treated with diethylstilbestrol (Fig 6). This phenomenon serves to emphasize that the same hormonal agent which under some circumstances can prove to be carcinogenic can also be shown to be oncolytic under other conditions. These opposing effects have been known for ionizing radiation for some time. This paradox warrants our full consideration.

More recently, advanced endometrial cancer has been shown to respond in about one third of the cases to massive doses of synthetic progestins (38,39). In addition, the suppression of endometrial carcinoma-in-situ as well as adenomatous hyperplasia of the endometrium by massive progestin therapy has been demonstrated (40). The view that these effects are mediated through the anti-estrogenic effects of the progestins is supported by numerous experimental studies. Pertinent to one of the main themes of this volume is the report of Nordqvist (18) that the in vitro progestin-binding capacity of biopsies from patients with endometrial carcinoma are frequently related to their clinical response to exogenous progestins.

It is interesting that the kidney should prove to be the site of a hormone-responsive tumor. Consideration of this possibility arose from the experimental induction of renal tumors by chronic estrogen administration in hamsters (41). In addition, the kidney is known to exhibit a sexual dimorphism in mice. These considerations have led to the use of progestins in the treatment of renal carcinoma in man (42). This then is another example of a clinical carry-over of basic animal studies in this ever-evolving field of steroid-related tumors.

REFERENCES

1. Velardo, J.T., In: Martini, L. and Pecile, A. (eds.), Hormonal Steroids, Vol. I, Academic Press, 1964, p.463.

2. Dorfman, R.I., In: Martini, L. and Pecile, A. (eds.), Hormonal Steroids, Vol. I, Academic Press, 1964, p.39.

3. Huggins, C. and Clark, P.J., J. Exp. Med. 72:747, 1940.

4. Courrier, R., Vitamins and Hormones, Vol. 8, Academic Press, 1950, p.179.

5. Hertz, R., Larsen, C.D. and Tullner, W.W., J. Nat. Cancer Inst. 8:123, 1947.

6. Mowszowicz, I., Bieber, D.E., Chung, K.W., Bullock, C.P. and Bardin, C.W., Endocrinology 95:1589, 1974.

7. Landau, R.L., Bergenstal, D.M., Lugibihl, K. and Kascht, M.E., J. Clin. Endocrinol. Metab. 15:1194, 1955.

8. Hertz, R. and Tullner, W.W., Proc. Soc. Exp. Biol. Med. 99: 451, 1958.

9. Dorfman, R.I., Endocrinology 42:7, 1948.

10. Bardin, C.W., Bullock, L.P., Sherins, R.J., Mowszowicz, I. and Blackborn, W.R., Recent Progr. Hormone Res. 29:65, 1973.

11. Bardin, C.W., Bullock, L., Schneider, G., Allison, J.E. and Stanley, A.J., Science 167:1136, 1970.

12. Ohno, S. and Lyon, M.F., Clin. Genet. 1:121, 1970.

13. Stanley, A.J., Gumbreck, L.G., Allison, L.E. and Easley, R.B., Recent Progr. Hormone Res. 29:43, 1973.

14. Gardner, W.U., Pfeiffer, C.A. and Trentin, J.J., In: Homburger, F. and Fishman, W.H. (eds.), Pathophysiology of Cancer, Ed. 2, Harper & Row, 1959, p.152.

15. Little, C.C., In: Homburger, F. and Fishman, W.H. (eds.), Pathophysiology of Cancer, Ed. 2, Harper & Row, 1959, p.127.

16. McGuire, W.L., Carbone, P.P. and Vollmer, E.P. (eds.), Estrogen Receptors in Human Breast Cancer, Raven Press, New York, 1975.

17. McGuire, W.L. and Julian, J.A., Cancer Res. 31:1440, 1971.

18. Nordqvist, S., Gynecol. Oncology 2:415, 1974.

19. Herbst, A.L., Ulfelder, U. and Poskanzer, D.C., New England J. Med. 284:878, 1971.

20. Herbst, A.L., Robboy, S.J., Scully, R.E. and Poskanzer, D.C., Am. J. Obstet. Gynec. 119:713, 1974.

21. Herbst, A.L., Poskanzer, D.C. and Robboy, S.J., New England J. Med. 292:334, 1975.

22. Lanier, A.P., Noller, K.L. and Dlecker, D.G., Mayo Clinic Proceedings 48:793, 1973.

23. Ulfelder, H., National Conference on Gynecol. Cancer, Sept., 1975, Cancer, In Press.

24. Heinonen, O.P., Cancer 31:573, 1973.

25. Hueper, W.C., Occupational Tumors and Allied Diseases, C.C. Thomas, Springfield, 1942.

26. Hertz, R., Int. J. Fert. 13:273, 1968.

27. Cutler, B.S., Forbes, A.D., Ingersoll, F.M. and Scully, R.E., New England J. Med. 287:628, 1972.

28. Hisaw, F.L. and Lendrum, F.C., Endocrinology 20:228, 1936.

29. Reagan, J.W., Gynecol. Oncology 2:144, 1974.

30. Smith, D.C. and Herrmann, W., Am. College of Obstet. Gynecol. District VIII, Los Angeles, Nov. 6, 1974.

31. Ostergaard, E., Proceedings of Int. College of Gynecol. and Obstet., Geneva, July 26, 1954, p.222.

32. Nissen, E.D. and Kent, D.R., Obstet. Gynec. 46:460, 1975.

33. Liddle, G.W., Island, D., Lance, E.M. and Harris, A.P., J. Clin. Endocrinol. 18:906, 1958.

34. Hertz, R., Pittman, J.A. and Graff, M.M., J. Clin. Endorinol. 16:705, 1956.

35. Fishman, L.M., Liddle, G.W., Island, D.P., Fleischer, N. and Kuchel, O., J. Clin. Endocrinol. 27:481, 1967.

36. Bergenstal, D.M., Hertz, R., Lipsett, M.D. and Moy, R.H., Ann. Int. Med. 53:672, 1960.

37. Hutter, A.M. and Kayhoe, D.E., Am. J. Med. 41:581, 1966.

38. Reifenstein, E., Gynecol. Oncology 2:377, 1974.

39. Kelley, R.M. and Baker, W.H., In: Pincus, G. and Vollmer, E.P. (eds.), Biological Activities of Steroids in Relation to Cancer, Academic Press, New York, 1960, p. 427.

40. Kistner, R.W., Cancer 18:1563, 1959.

41. Kirkman, H.W., Nat. Cancer Inst. Monogr. 1:1, 1959.

42. Bloom, H.J.G., In: Stoll, D.A. (ed.), Endocrine Therapy in Malignant Disease, Chapter 18, Saunders, Philadelphia, 1972, p. 339.

THE ETIOLOGY OF BREAST CANCER

Marvin A. Rich, Philip Furmanski, Charles M. McGrath, Justin McCormick, Jose Russo, and Herbert Soule

Biology Department
Michigan Cancer Foundation
Detroit, Michigan

INTRODUCTION

A dominant focus of the research programs at our own and other laboratories remains the identification and characterization of the populations at high risk to breast cancer. The goal: the early detection of the disease and, ultimately, its biological control.

Breast cancer is the leading cause of cancer deaths in women. It is demonstrably polymorphic in nature and its cause is likely polyfactorial.

The incidence of breast cancer varies widely from one population to another. The frequency of the disease in Northern European and North American women, for example, is much higher than in Oriental or Latin American women (Table 1). Demographic and laboratory studies have suggested, with varying degrees of certainty, that many general and specific factors (Table 2) may contribute to the development of breast cancer. The role of viruses in this process has held the attention of our own laboratories for some time. The origin of our interest lies in the fact that mammary cancer in experimental animals can be induced by viruses, and by the discovery that similar virus particles are present in human milk, in human mammary epithelial cells, and in cell lines derived from human breast cancers.

TABLE 1

Breast Cancer Death Rates

	Deaths per 100,000 per year*
Dominican Republic	2.9
China	3.7
Japan	4.0
Mexico	4.2
Hindus (of Bombay)	6.0
Yugoslavia	8.1
Hong Kong	8.4
Italy	16.1
Norway	16.8
Parsis (of Bombay)	18.2
U.S.A.	21.9
New Zealand	23.1
South Africa	23.1
Netherlands	26.5

*Age adjusted, 1967 base.

TABLE 2

Factors Affecting the Incidence of Breast Cancer

Hormone Status	Child Bearing Experience
Diet	Socioeconomic Status
Body Dimensions	Viruses
Family History of Cancer	

THE MOUSE MAMMARY TUMOR VIRUS (MuMTV)

The etiologic role of viruses in the mammary tumors of mice was first demonstrated forty years ago by John Bittner (1). As in humans, mammary cancer in the mouse is not a uniform disease. Both the susceptibility to mammary tumor viruses and the subsequent influence of hormones on the development of the disease vary widely from strain to strain.

The classic studies of Bittner established that mammary cancers in mice could be caused by a virus which in turn could be transmitted through nursing milk. These viruses are classified as type B oncornaviruses (Fig 1). Their genetic information is coded by a 70S RNA. They possess reverse transcriptase (RNA-dependent DNA polymerase) enzymes and biophysical properties similar to those of the other oncornaviruses known to induce neoplasia, in several host species.

MuMTV is an endogenous virus of mice - that is, the nucleic acid information for MuMTV is contained in the genome of every cell of the host. Since all mice do not develop mammary cancers, it is evident that every mouse with the potential (genetic information) to synthesize MuMTV does not express this potential without the further intervention of genetic, hormonal or other environmental influences. Nevertheless, a relationship firmly and reliably established between human breast cancer and specific viruses would, beyond answering the theoretical question of breast cancer etiology, open doors to the development of techniques for the very early detection and perhaps the prevention of the disease.

VIRUS IN HUMAN MILK

It is known that there are at least two routes of natural transmission for the mouse mammary tumor virus - by way of the milk and by vertical transmission through viral genomic information integrated into, and transmitted by, the germ cells.

The development of mammary cancer in mice varies considerably as a function both of the mode of the transmission and of the hormonal status of the host strain. However, virus particles and their antigens can usually be found in the milk of all infected mice that ultimately develop mammary tumors.

Since human populations with relatively high incidence of breast cancer had been identified, a search in human milk for viruses similar to MuMTV seemed appropriate.

The Parsi Community of Bombay seemed particularly suitable for these studies. The Parsi migrated from Persia to India in the

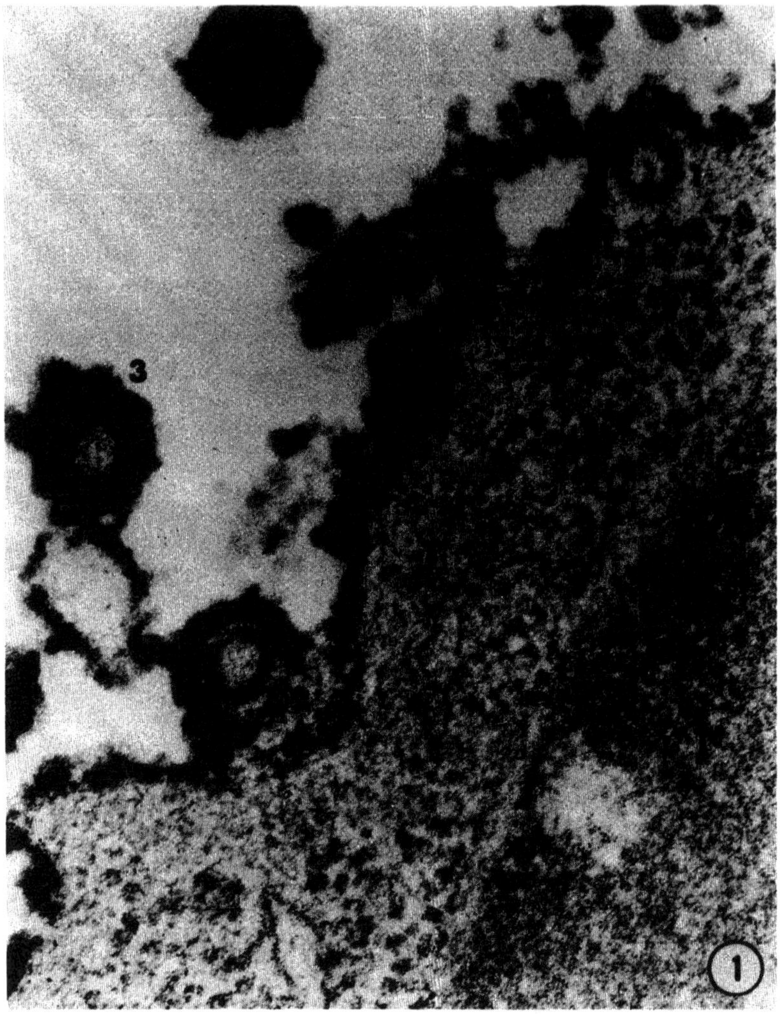

Fig 1. Murine mammary tumor cell synthesizing type B oncornavirus particles. 1 and 2 are virus particles in different stages of budding; 3 is a free, immature type B particle; N is the cell nucleus. X 150,000.

seventh century and as a consequence of their strict prohibition against inter-marriage constitute a population that has been inbred for almost fifteen hundred years.

While the overall incidence of breast cancer in Parsi women is somewhat less than that in European women, it is three times higher than in the non-Parsi, Hindu population of Bombay. Almost fifty percent of all the cancers seen in Parsi women are breast cancers.

In this (2) and subsequent studies on other populations (3), virus particles with the characteristics of known animal oncornaviruses were observed in the milk of these women. These particles were morphologically similar to MuMTV.

Since the available epidemiological information suggested that the general population could be divided into high- and low-risk sub-sets, an attempt was begun by several laboratories* to determine if women at higher risk to breast cancer had detectably higher levels of oncornavirus in their milk.

Unfortunately, the tools which have been available for the detection and the quantification of oncornaviruses have proved less than satisfactory when applied to the routine, large scale testing of complex body fluids.

Three avenues of approach are available for the detection of these viruses: they are (a) morphological, (b) biochemical, and (c) immunological.

Several electron microscopic studies have described the distribution of virus-like particles in negatively stained preparations of human milk. It has been shown, however, that exposure to human milk could destroy the morphological integrity of exogenously added MuMTV (4), and further that human milks contain membranous vesicles and casein micelles which can be mistaken for oncornaviruses in negatively stained preparations.

In collaboration with Dr. Karl Maramorosch (Rutgers University), we have shown (5) that the unambiguous electron detection of virus in milk requires thin sectioning techniques. Using human milk seeded with known quantities of an animal RNA tumor virus, differential centrifugation techniques were devised for the isolation and quantitation of these viruses.

The discovery of reverse transcriptase and its specific association with RNA tumor viruses (6,7) suggested its use in an

---

*With the support of the National Cancer Institute, the Michigan Cancer Foundation has organized an extensive human milk collecting network which annually monitors more than 70,000 obstetrical deliveries in the metropolitan Detroit area. This resource system provides milk specimens for our own research program, and has for the last two years, been providing human milk samples to the National Cancer Institute for distribution to other laboratories.

enzyme assay for the detection of such viruses in human milk (8). Other studies on the distribution of virus particles in human milk suggested however, that human milk might contain factors that would obviate the reliable detection of reverse transcriptase. Our own work (9) has identified one such inhibitor as ribonuclease. In one series of human milks examined, 22 of 25 milks contained sufficient ribonuclease to completely mask the activity of more than 10^8 virus particles per ml. It is possible therefore, that oncornaviruses in human milk and in other body fluids, can be detected by reverse transcriptase assay only when their titer is very high, or when the RNAse level of the milk is correspondingly low. Hence, the variation in oncornavirus content of human milk, as determined by reverse transcriptase assay, in studies aimed at correlating virus content with risk to breast cancer, may actually reflect not the absolute quantity of virus in the milk, but instead an inverse measure of the level of RNAse which the milks contained.

While it appears certain that these virions are present in some human milks, the true distribution of oncornavirus in human milk, and the relationship of this factor to the incidence of breast cancer, remains to be clarified.

To accomplish this, we have been examining alternate methods for virus detection in human milk. A useful approach appears to be a specific radioimmunoassay for virus antigens. Such assays have been developed for many of the animal oncornaviruses, including MuMTV. The requirements for such an assay include a highly purified protein isolated from the virus particle, and a high titered, specific antiserum reactive to it.

Since the membranous vesicles, casein micelles and fat globules in human milk interfere with the purification of virus particles, our approach to the isolation of virus proteins has relied instead on the preparation of viral cores.

When oncornaviruses are disrupted by ether and detergent treatment the RNA- and protein-containing viral cores can be separated from the virus coat proteins by density gradient centrifugation (The core has a higher density than does the intact virus). The resulting shift in density which occurs during core preparation is thus used to eliminate contaminating proteins. It has been shown that such sub-virus cores can be prepared from the virus particles in human milk (10).

With this technique we have isolated a protein which is associated with the oncornavirus-like particle in human milk. This protein is present in reverse transcriptase positive milks, and absent in negative milks. Its distribution in density gradients of core preparations coincides with the core-containing bands and their reverse transcriptase activity (11). It is noteworthy that the core protein isolated from human milk is electrophoretically identical to the major core protein of MuMTV (27,000 daltons).

Several reports suggest a relationship between MuMTV and human breast cancers. These have been based on both immunological (12) and molecular hybridization techniques (13). It has been suggested further, that a candidate human breast cancer virus (14) similarly shares some homology with MuMTV. Whether these homologies are a function of the major core protein remains to be determined.

It should be noted that the availability of a radioimmunoassay, which does not require the maintenance of an intact virus structure, and does not depend on the detection of a labile enzyme activity, would permit the detection of oncornavirus in body fluids and tissues other than milk and would thus permit the extension of these studies beyond the lactating population.

VIRUS IN NORMAL HUMAN MAMMARY EPITHELIAL CELLS

It is likely that the virus-like particles found in human milk originate from the normal, milk secreting, epithelial cells of the breast, and that these cells may be better indicators of the virological status of the human host than is milk itself. These cells could serve not only as a potential virus source, but also as a substrate for infectivity studies.

Since human milk was known to contain such cells, we attempted to use this fluid as a source for initiating cultures of mammary epithelial cells. We found that the cells in the milk of actively lactating donors were present in very low concentration (generally fewer than 10^4 cells per sample), and that most of the cells were damaged and would not grow. When sequential samples of milk from single donors were examined, we observed that a peak in the cell concentration of milks occurred just after the onset of weaning, when the volume of secreted breast fluid is drastically reduced. These cells, when placed in culture with the addition of autologous serum develop into monolayers of growing epithelial cells (15,16) (Fig 2).

Cells grown in culture from human post-weaning fluids retain the ultrastructural features of normal mammary epithelium (17). The cells are interconnected by a network of true desmosomes, possess microvilli, and a highly developed Golgi apparatus with substantial quantities of secretory material in the cisternae and vesicles.

Cells from some human donors exhibit evidence of oncornavirus synthesis (15). The low levels of virus synthesis and the restricted

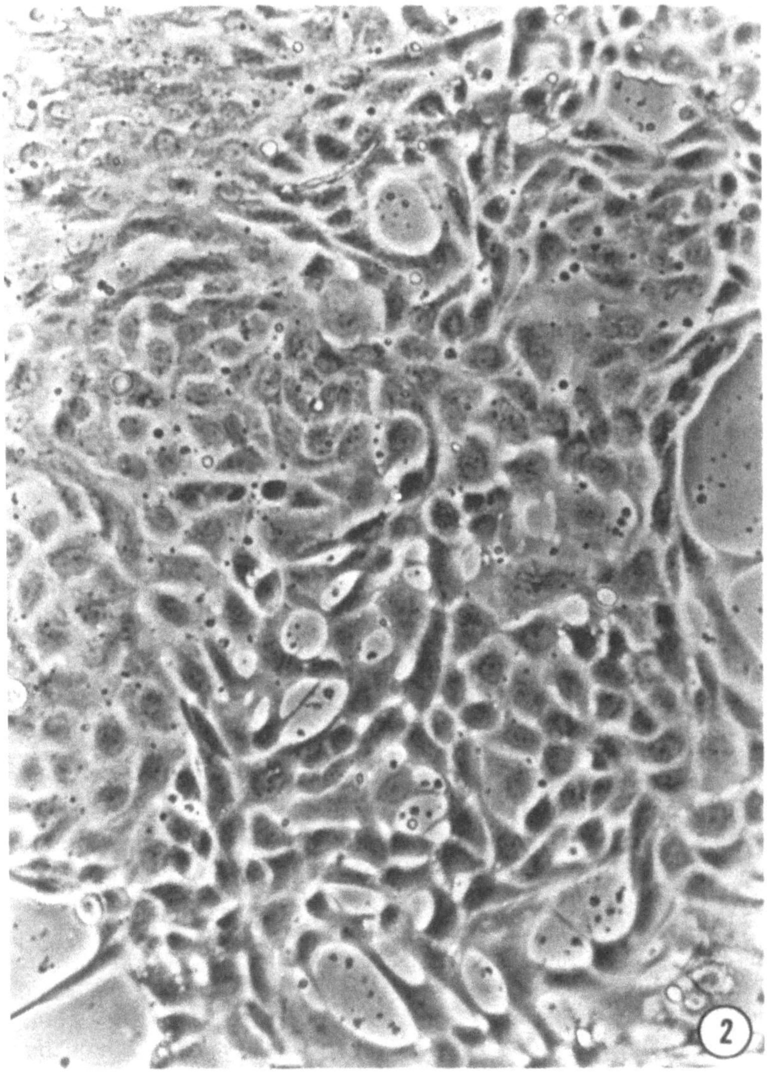

Fig 2. Culture of normal human mammary epithelial cells derived from a post-weaning breast fluid.

growth potential of these cells in culture have, to date, limited our ability to further characterize the virus-like particle synthesized by normal human mammary epithelial cells and to compare this particle with those found in human milk and human breast cancers. It is anticipated that more sensitive immunological and nucleic acid hybridization methods will facilitate such efforts.

VIRUS IN HUMAN BREAST CANCER CELLS

While work is underway to develop methods for the reliable and reproducible quantification of human milk virions, it is also necessary to examine the biological properties of these virions. Many of the techniques required for viral characterization can only be applied in vitro. The development of in vitro systems for the isolation and propagation of candidate human breast cancer viruses represents another major effort of our laboratories.

We have reported the development of a permanent cell line (MCF-7) from a pleural effusion in a patient with a malignant adenocarcinoma of the breast (18). This cell line has been extensively characterized; it has been shown to be human, to be derived from mammary epithelium, and to possess several characteristics of malignant cells. The results are summarized in Table 3.

MCF-7 cells synthesize a particle (734B) with all of the characteristics of the known oncornaviruses (14). The particle, which shares no identity with mammalian leukemia viruses has a density of 1.17 gms/cc, contains a true reverse transcriptase, and 70S RNA. Particle synthesis is however, slightly restricted, with only transient, low level virus production observed in routine cell culture passages of MCF-7.

To define the biological role of this agent it was necessary to confirm its species of origin. Such determinations are based on the fact that endogenous oncornaviruses of any species are coded by the DNA genome of the native species. Unrelated species do not carry the same coding sequence in their DNA, and consequently, one can expect the viral genome (or a DNA copy of it) to hybridize with the DNA of the species of origin but not with the DNA of unrelated species.

Our results to date suggest that at least some 734B sequences are coded by the DNA genome of human cells and not by non-human cells, and suggest, therefore that 734B is a human endogenous virus.

In the mouse mammary cancer system, virus is found in milk, in cultured cells derived from tumor, and in breast tumors. Might we expect the same in man? The search in human breast tumors for 734B, or its genomic image has been initiated. In our experiments to date, we have observed the specific hybridization of 734B complementary DNA probes to RNA's from the breast tumors of six patients. No hybridization was observed between 734B probes and the RNA of normal human placenta or liver cells (26).

What is the relationship between the etiology of breast cancer in man and in the mouse? Neutralization of mouse mammary tumor

TABLE 3

MCF-7 - A Human, Mammary, Epithelial Cell Line

Humanness Established by:

1. Karyotype[1] (18,19)
2. Cell surface antigenicity*
3. The human isozyme of glucose-6-phosphate dehydrogenase
4. Ribosomal RNA of a molecular weight characteristic of the human species (18)

Derivation from Mammary Epithelium Established by:

1. High affinity estrogen receptor (20)
2. High affinity progesterone receptor (21)
3. α-Lactalbumin (human milk protein) synthesis (22)
4. Ultrastructure (23)

Malignancy Suggested by:

1. Growth in soft agar (24)
2. Agglutination by concanavalin A (24)
3. Tumor formation in nude mice (25)

virus by sera of human breast cancer patients (27), and the lymphocyte migration studies of Black and Moore and their associates (12), suggest that certain human breast cancers share antigenic components with mouse mammary tumor virus. Some cross hybridization between RNA from human breast tumors and DNA probe prepared from mouse mammary tumor virus have also been reported (13).

We are asking the direct question: Does the candidate human breast cancer virus, 734B, share common components with mouse mammary tumor viruses? The 734B particle does show some homology with MuMTV. MCF-7 cells which are actively producing 734B particles exhibit a low but reproducible level of specific fluorescence with

*Our studies were carried out in collaboration with Drs. Cyrus Stulberg and Ward Peterson, Children's Hospital and Research Institute, Detroit, Mi.

antiserum to MuMTV structural proteins, and non-virus producing MCF-7 cells do not (14). Labelled 734B proteins bind specifically to immunoadsorbent columns prepared with anti-MuMTV sera. This cross-reactivity appears to be at least part of a function of the major core protein of MuMTV. The candidate human breast cancer virus and MuMTV have proteins of 27-28,000 molecular weight, and it is this protein of 734B which is the major species bound to the anti-MuMTV immunoabsorbent columns (28). It should be noted that a major MuMTV protein, -- gp 52 - is absent in 734B.

Final proof that 734B is in fact a human breast cancer virus will require the determination of its specific biological activity. Is 734B capable of transforming normal cells into neoplastic cells? In the mouse, such experiments were comparatively easy. However, the same experimental methods are not available for human studies and proof of the virus' oncogenic potential will perforce need to be indirect.

Following inoculation with 734B, the demonstration of neoplastic transformation or its precursive characteristics in previously normal cells would, for example, provide substantial support for this oncogenic potential of 734B. Similarly the inoculation of 734B into non-human mammals could be used to directly measure its tumorigenic potential.

Whether or not the attainment of these goals ultimately permits an unequivocal demonstration of a viral causality, the specific association of such viruses or their antigens with human breast cancers may nevertheless, provide useful tools for early detection of the primary and recurrent disease. With respect to the latter, it will be of interest to determine if such associated viral antigens or their absence are involved in that facet of the tumor-host relationship which is determinant for recurring or metastatic diseases.

ACKNOWLEDGMENT

Authors' work described in this report has been supported by National Institutes of Health Contract #NO1-CP-33347, the Suzanne Korman Morton Memorial Fund of the Michigan Cancer Foundation and an institutional grant from the United Foundation of metropolitan Detroit.

REFERENCES

1. Bittner, J.J., Science 84:162, 1936.

2. Moore, D.H., J. Charney, B. Kramarski, E.Y. Lasfargues, N.H. Sarkar, M.H. Brennan, H.N. Burrows, S.M. Sirsat, J.C. Paymaster and A.B. Vaidya, Nature 229:611, 1971.

3. Feller, W.F. and H.C. Chopra, Cancer 28:1425, 1971.

4. Sarkar, N.H., J. Charney, A.S. Dion and D.H. Moore, Cancer Res. 33:626, 1973.

5. Maramorosch, K., H. Hirumi, M. Kimura, R. Rich, P. Furmanski and M.A. Rich, Submitted for Publication.

6. Baltimore, D., Nature 226:1209, 1970.

7. Temin, H. and S. Mizutani, Nature 226:1211, 1971.

8. Schlom, J., S. Spiegelman and D.H. Moore, Nature 231:97, 1971.

9. McCormick, J.J., L.J. Larson and M.A. Rich, Nature 251: 737, 1974.

10. Feldman, S.P., Schlom, J. and S. Spiegelman, Proc. Nat. Acad. Sci., U.S.A. 70:1976, 1973.

11. Furmanski, P., C.P. Loeckner, C.P., Longley, C., L.J. Larson and M.A. Rich, Submitted for Publication.

12. Black, M.M., P.H. Moore, B. Shore, R.E. Zachran and M.P. Leis, Cancer Res. 34:1054, 1974.

13. Spiegelman, S., Axel, R. and J. Schlom, J. National Cancer Inst. 48:1205, 1972.

14. McGrath, C.M., P.M. Grant, H.D. Soule, T. Glancy and M.A. Rich, Nature 252:247, 1974.

15. Furmanski, P., C. Longley, D. Fouchey, R. Rich and M.A. Rich, J. National Cancer Inst. 52:975, 1974.

16. Furmanski, P., C. Longley, D. Fouchey, R. Rich and M.A. Rich, Fed. Proc. 33:753, 1974.

17. Russo, J., P. Furmanski and M.A. Rich, Am. J. Anat. 142: 221, 1975.

18. Soule, H.D., J. Vasquez, A. Long, S. Albert and M.J. Brennan, J. National Cancer Inst. 51:1409, 1973.

19. Nelson-Rees, W., R. Flandermayer and P. Hawthorne, Science 184:1093, 1974.

20. Brooks, S., E. Locke and H. Soule, J. Biol. Chem. 248: 6251, 1973.

21. Lippman, M.E., G. Bolan and K. Huff, Nature 258:29, 1975.

22. Rose, H.N. and C.M. McGrath, Science 190:673, 1975.

23. Arnold, W.J., H.D. Soule and J. Russo, In Vitro 10:62, 1975.

24. Voyles, B.A., H. Soule and C.M. McGrath, In Vitro 10:389, 1975.

25. Russo, J., C.M. McGrath, I. Russo and M.A. Rich, III Inter. Symp. on Detection and Prevention of Cancer, New York, 1976.

26. Das, M.R., C.M. McGrath and M.A. Rich, Unpublished Results.

27. Charney, J. and D.H. Moore, Nature 229:627, 1971.

28. McGrath, C.M., P. Furmanski, H. Soule, P. Grant, C. Longley and M.A. Rich, Proc. Am. Assoc. Cancer Res. 16:164, 1975.

SELECTING ENDOCRINE THERAPY IN BREAST CANCER

W.L. McGuire, K.B. Horwitz and M. De La Garza

Health Science Center
University of Texas
San Antonio, Texas 78284

In estrogen target tissues and hormone-dependent tumors, the steroid enters the cells and binds to a cytoplasmic protein called the estrogen receptor (ER). The steroid-receptor complex then migrates to the nuclei, where it initiates the biochemical events characteristic of estrogen stimulation. Since ER is absent in tissues not responsive to estrogen, studies have been designed to show whether ER in human breast cancer might be used to identify those patients likely to respond to endocrine therapy.

Data on 436 clinical trials contributed from a dozen centers around the world now clearly indicate that if a patient's tumor does not contain ER, there is virtually no chance of tumor regression following endocrine therapy. When their tumors have ER, 55-60% of patients respond to endocrine therapy, so that this single piece of data, when coupled with available clinical prognostic factors such as menopausal status, disease-free interval, site of the dominant lesion, and especially response to previous hormonal therapies, should permit the practicing oncologist to select or reject endocrine therapy with confidence. If our hypothesis involving the use of the progesterone receptor (PgR) as a marker of endocrine responsive tumors is supported, then the 40% of ER+ tumors which will be endocrine resistant will also be identifiable and a large number of patients would be spared unrewarding therapies.

INTRODUCTION

The human mammary gland is exquisitely sensitive to a number of hormones, and one would predict that tumors arising by malignant transformation of mammary gland cells retain these hormone controls.

Indeed, the first demonstration of the regression of metastatic breast cancer in response to ovariectomy was made 78 years ago (1). Unfortunately, only 30% of such metastatic tumors are responsive, and usually respond equally well to adrenalectomy or hypophysectomy (2). Since little is known of the complex hormonal interrelationships involved in tumor growth, tumors are classified simply as "hormone dependent".

Target tissues for any hormone contain specific receptors for that hormone - - cytoplasmic proteins for the steroids, and surface membrane molecules for polypeptides and some others. Hormone dependent tumors also contain receptors, but it now appears that independent, or autonomous, tumors often may not (3). These findings, which will be discussed, have led to the following hypothesis:

1. Normal mammary cells contain cytoplasmic or membrane receptor sites for each of the hormones known to influence growth and function of the mammary gland. These receptor sites are responsible for the initial interaction between the hormone and the cell, and trigger the biochemical events characteristic for the particular hormone.

2. When malignant transformation occurs, the cell may retain all or part of the normal population of receptor sites. If the malignant cell retains receptors, its growth and function is potentially capable of being regulated by the hormonal environment as in a normal cell and such tumors would be responsive to endocrine therapy.

3. If specific receptors are lost from the tumor this may indicate that the tumor is endocrine resistant, and would be unresponsive to endocrine manipulation.

Only estrogen receptors have thus far been studied with respect to this hypothesis. The preferential uptake of radioactive estrogen by target tissues and endocrine responsive tumors, was demonstrated in vivo and in vitro in the years following 1959; endocrine resistant tumors were less active (4-10). The discovery of the specific receptor for estrogen in these responsive tissues explained the preferential uptake of the hormone and also suggested that tumors could be assayed for receptor, to predict hormone dependence.

Estrogen Receptor in Human Breast Tumors

The properties of the estrogen receptor (ER) as determined in induced hormone dependent rat tumors have now been found in human mammary tumor cytosols as well (11). Two of these properties are employed in our laboratory to quantify ER in human breast cancer specimens obtained at surgery (12,13). The first is the high affinity binding of ^{3}H-estradiol, evaluated by equilibrating cytosol with various low concentrations of labelled hormone and then removing the unbound hormone with dextran-coated charcoal. Scatchard plots of the binding data show that the receptor, if present, has a very high affinity binding component (Kd $< 1 \times 10^{-10}$M). By direct extrapolation, the amount of this component can be determined. The second property, the sedimentation of receptor primarily at 8S in low salt sucrose gradients, is employed to confirm the results of the charcoal assay by an independent method. Because part of the 4S binding peak may also be due to specific receptor, a parallel gradient is always run with a 100-fold excess of unlabelled diethylstilbestrol to measure any nonspecific binding components.

With these techniques, we are in a position to explore Jensen's original suggestion that the presence of ER in a human breast tumor might indicate that the tumor was hormone dependent and could be made to regress by appropriate endocrine manipulation (6). To this date our laboratory has assayed ER in 750 human breast tumors for eventual correlation with response to endocrine therapy (14).

We find that the values in primary tumors range from 0 to about 1000 femtomoles per mg of cytosol protein. (The level of sensitivity in the two methods is such that a value of less than 3 is essentially equivalent to 0 and is considered a negative assay). Positive ER values (≥ 3) are found in 70% of primary specimens and 58% of metastatic specimens. We have previously speculated that the wide range of values apparent in our results is due to a combination of factors, including: a) variations in epithelial vs. stromal content of the tumors, b) the degree of dedifferentiation of the tumor, and c) the patient's endogenous estrogen levels, since endogenous estradiol would occupy ER sites and make them unavailable for assay. This last point may at least partially explain why the highest values for tumor ER are seen in postmenopausal patients.

CLINICAL CORRELATION

A number of other laboratories (using a variety of techniques) have also assayed ER in breast tumor specimens. Data on clinical response to endocrine therapy are now available in many of these cases. To correlate these data an international workshop sponsored by the Breast Cancer Task Force of the National Cancer Institute was held in Bethesda, Maryland on July 18-19, 1974. Details of both ER assay procedures and clinical evaluation criteria were examined, and 436 treatment trials in 380 patients were ultimately accepted. We will provide a brief overview of the data presented at that meeting, indicating the current status of ER assays in predicting response to endocrine therapies in patients with metastatic breast cancer. For details, the reader should consult the specific manuscripts and summary chapter published in the conference proceedings (15).

Response to Endocrine Therapy

1. Extramural Review - Since the organizing committee for this conference felt that clinical response data was as critical as the ER assay data itself, it was arranged that participating institutions could request an extramural review of their case material. Prior to the conference, eight institutions were visited by two oncologists (Mary E. Sears and George C. Escher) and a total of 531 treatment trials in 453 patients were reviewed by the following criteria:

Objective remission was defined as a decrease in size of at least 50% of the measurable lesions by more than 50%, while other lesions remained unchanged and no new lesions appeared. As the standard basis for determining the size of a lesion, the product of the two longest perpendicular diameters of the lesions was used. In osteolytic metastasis, evidence of healing upon roentgenography was necessary, again without increase in size or number of destructive lesions. Osteoblastic metastasis as the only measurable lesion was not an acceptable criterion for the study. In cases with multiple skin lesions, which often are impossible to measure with accuracy, photographs served as the means for evaluation of response. Neither the healing of an ulcerating lesion nor the clearing of pleural effusion was accepted as objective evidence of remission. Complete agreement between the investigators' and the reviewers' evaluations was attained in 442 of the 531 reviewed treatment trials. There were only 17 instances of total disagreement, but a relatively larger number in which the intramural evaluation could not be supported because of inadequate documentation.

2. Clincial Correlation of ER and Response to Endocrine Therapy - The 436 treatment trials in 380 patients evaluated by the extramural review team are summarized in Table 1.

Surgical Ablation (Castration, Adrenalectomy, Hypophysectomy)

Thirty-three percent of 201 treatment trials resulted in objective tumor regressions. Of the 94 trials in patients with negative tumor ER values, only 8 (8%) were successful, whereas 59 (55%) of the 107 trials in patients with positive tumor ER values succeeded. Patients with borderline tumor ER values had a 30% response rate.

TABLE 1

Objective Breast Tumor Regressions According to ER Assay and Type of Therapy as Judged by Extramural Review[a]

Therapy	ER+	ER-
Adrenalectomy	32/66	4/33
Castration	25/33	4/53
Hypophysectomy	2/8	0/8
TOTAL:	59/107 = 55%	8/94 = 8%
Androgen	12/26	2/24
Estrogen	37/57	5/58
Glucocorticoid	2/2	-
TOTAL:	51/85 = 60%	7/82 = 8%

[a]Adapted from reference 15.

Additive Therapy (Pharmacological Doses of Estrogens, Androgens, and Glucocorticoids)

Thirty-four percent of 167 trials resulted in objective tumor regressions. Of the 82 trials in patients with negative tumor ER values, 7 (8%) were successful, whereas 51 (60%) of the 85 trials in patients with positive tumor ER values succeeded.

There remains little doubt that estrogen receptor values can be helpful in predicting the results of endocrine therapy for metastatic breast cancer. It is clear that if a patient has a negative tumor ER values the chances of tumor regression in response to endocrine therapy are minimal. A large number of patients can thus be spared unrewarding major endocrine ablative therapy if ER assays are performed routinely. When the tumor ER value is positive the response to endocrine therapy is 55-60%. This single piece of evidence when coupled with available clinical prognostic factors such as menopausal status, disease-free interval, site of dominant lesion, and especially response to previous hormonal therapies should permit the practicing oncologist to select or reject endocrine therapy with relative confidence. Our concern now is to identify the 40% of ER+ tumors which have lost their hormone dependence, so that these patients can be spared unrewarding therapies.

Progesterone Receptors in Human Breast Cancer

The presence of ER in malignant cells is evidence that at least part of the normal control system remains intact. However, since binding to receptors is only an early step in hormone action, it is possible that in ER+ tumors where endocrine manipulations fail, the lesion is at a later step. An ideal marker of an endocrine responsive tumor would therefore be a measurable product of hormone action rather than the initial binding step. Because in estrogen target tissues, the synthesis of progesterone receptor (PgR) depends on the action of estrogen, we investigated the possibility that PgR might be such a marker (16). If so, it would be expected that PgR would be rare in tumors which lack ER. The presence of PgR in tumors containing ER would indicate that the tumors are capable of synthesizing at least one end product under estrogen regulation and that the tumors remain endocrine responsive. Tumors with ER but no PgR would be resistant to endocrine therapy.

We have used 8S binding of the synthetic progestin ^{3}H-R5020 (Roussel UCLAF) in sucrose gradients to identify PgR in human breast cancer tissue, rather than resorting to indirect differential competition studies. Excess nonradioactive progesterone or R5020 completely inhibits the 8S ^{3}H-R5020 binding, whereas hydrocortisone, dexamethasone, or estradiol do not compete effectively (17). We have now determined PgR and ER in more than 300 human mammary tumors. PgR is present in only 8% of the tumors lacking ER. Of the ER+ tumors, 62% had PgR. This distribution is similar to the response rate to endocrine therapies for ER+ and ER- tumors and is consistent with the hypothesis that PgR may be a marker for hormone dependence. Of course, confirmation of this hypothesis requires direct correlation of the presence of PgR and objectively defined clinical remission. Our preliminary clinical data is encouraging (18). If further clinical correlations support our hypothesis, the presence of PgR will show that at least a part of the hormone response system is functional, thus providing a more accurate marker of hormone dependence.

ACKNOWLEDGMENTS

These studies were supported in part by the USPHS CA-11378, CB-23862, and the American Cancer Society, BC23D. We thank Dr. J. P. Raynaud and Roussel UCLAF for the generous gift of R5020 and Dennis Perotta for his expert technical assistance.

REFERENCES

1. Beatson, G.T., Lancet 2:104 & 162, 1896.

2. Dao, T.L., Ann. Rev. Med. 23:1, 1972.

3. McGuire, W.L., G.C. Chamness, M.E. Costlow and R.E. Shepherd, Metabolism 23:75, 1974.

4. Folca, P.J., R.F. Glascock and W.T. Irvine, Lancet 2:796, 1961.

5. Glascock, R.F. and W.G. Hoekstra, Biochem. J. 72:673, 1959.

6. Jensen, E.V., E.R. DeSombre and P.W. Jungblut, In: Wissler, R.W., T.L. Dao and S. Wood (eds.), Endogenous Factors Influencing Host-Tumor Balance, University of Chicago Press, Chicago, 1967, p.15.

7. Jensen, E.V. and H.I. Jacobson, In: Pincus, G. and E.P. Vollmer (eds.), Biological Activities of Steroids in Relation to Cancer, Academic Press, New York, 1960, p.161.

8. King, R.J.B., J. Gordon, D.M. Cowan and D.R. Inman, J. Endocrinol. 36:139, 1966.

9. Mobbs, B.G., J. Endocrinol. 36:409, 1966.

10. Terenius, L., Cancer Research 28:328, 1968.

11. McGuire, W.L. and M. De La Garza, J. Clin. Endocrinol. Metab. 36:548, 1973.

12. McGuire, W.L., J. Clin. Invest. 52:73, 1973.

13. McGuire, W.L. and M. De La Garza, J. Clin. Endocrinol. Metab. 37:986, 1973.

14. McGuire, W.L., O.H. Pearson and A. Segaloff, In: McGuire, W.L., P.P. Carbone and E.P. Vollmer (eds.), Estrogen Receptor in Human Breast Cancer, Raven Press, New York, 1975, p.17.

15. McGuire, W.L., P.P. Carbone, M.E. Sears and G.C. Escher, In: McGuire, W.L., P.P. Carbone and E.P. Vollmer (eds.), Estrogen Receptor in Human Breast Cancer, Raven Press, New York, 1975, p.1.

16. McGuire, W.L., G.C. Chamness, M.E. Costlow and K.B. Horwitz, In: Levey, G.S. (ed.), Modern Pharmacology, Marcel Dekker, Inc., New York, 1975, In Press.

17. Horwitz, K.B. and W.L. McGuire, Steroids 25:497, 1975.

18. Horwitz, K.B., W.L. McGuire, O.H. Pearson and A. Segaloff, Science 189:726, 1975.

THE METABOLISM OF STEROID HORMONES IN BREAST CANCER: A REAPPRAISAL

S.C. Brooks

Department of Biochemistry
Wayne State University, School of Medicine
Detroit, Michigan

MacMahon (1), Lemon (2) and Smith and Smith (3) have emphasized that abnormal ovarian function or steroid metabolism not modified by pregnancy in early life, may well be implicated in human breast cancer etiology. Wynder (4) and Dao (5) have pointed toward an etiological role for estrogen metabolism and nutritionally-conditioned alteration of estrogen metabolism in breast cancer, as also have Stocks (6) and Hems (7). The study of steroid excretion patterns in women with breast cancer (or prior to the onset of the disease) is further recommended by Bulbrook's observations in the women of Guernsey (8). Furthermore, there is some evidence (9) that at least part of the genetic predisposition of certain mouse strains is the result of genetically-determined ovarian function. These are but a few of the reports, published in the past decade, that pertain to steroid hormone metabolism in mammary cancer. However, before reappraising the data in this field it may be helpful to summarize what is now known of the fate of steroid hormones in the mammal.

FACTORS INVOLVED IN STEROID HORMONE HOMEOSTASIS

In women steroid hormone homeostasis is governed by many factors, several of which fluctuate with the hormonal milieu, age and the level of induction of certain enzymes involved in peripheral steroid metabolism. Both of the steroid secreting endocrine organs in the female, the ovary and the adrenal cortex, display decreased hormone secretion patterns with age. The ovary, of course, secretes estrogens, androgens and progestins in a cyclic fashion. These steroids are secreted in the unconjugated and sulfate form (10-12).

Once in the circulation steroid hormones are available to various tissues, including target organs, which actively metabolize the molecule. Certain target tissues metabolize steroids to active forms which bind to specific receptors prior to their nuclear uptake. Specific examples of this steroid potentiating metabolism are the oxidation and reduction of androst-5-ene-3β-ol-17-one (DHEA) to 5α-androstan-3-one-17β-ol (DHT) in skin adnexa (13,14) and the reduction of testosterone to DHT in prostate (15), and anterior pituitary (16) tissues. At the present time data indicate that this activation of steroid hormones by target tissues has little if any systemic effect. Responsive tissues may also "deactivate" specific steroid hormones <u>in situ</u> though oxidative processes such as the formation of estrone from 17β-estradiol (uterus, 17,18) or cortisone from cortisol (lymphocytes or fibroblasts, 19) and through the formation of estrogen sulfate esters which is characteristic of cycling porcine uterus (20).

Paraendocrine activity has been reported for hepatic and adipose tissues, particularly with respect to the aromatization of plasma androgens to estrogens (21-23). Although these pathways would be expected to contribute little to the level of plasma estrogens in the premenopausal woman, after menopause a significant portion of the plasma estrogens may be synthesized from circulating androgens. Such a phenomena would be expected to play a role in postmenopausal breast cancer.

Hepatic involvement in steroid hormone homeostasis has long been established. The biliary, urinary, and plasma concentrations of certain liver-formed steroid metabolites have been shown to vary in diseased states. For example, in chronic liver cirrhosis there is an interruption of the enterohepatic circulation resulting in decreased estrogen "deactivation". Such a situation not only results in less biliary excretion of the estrogens and their conjugates but this disease brings about a decrease in the 2-hydroxylation of estrogens (24) and a drop in the formation of estriol as well (24). Since these hydroxylated metabolites have been considered as "deactivated" estrogens, this metabolic abberation has been characterized in men by the appearance of gynaecomastia (25). Other experiments which support the concept of hepatic involvement in estrogen "deactivation" have been carried out with CCl_4-damaged liver, in which animals the apparent estrogen activity was greatly increased (26).

Principally the liver is capable of the reduction of A- or B-ring of neutral steroids thereby forming the 5α- or 5β-androstane or -pregnane compounds (27). In addition hepatic tissue (like many other tissues) contains active steroid dehydrogenases which interconvert hydroxyls and ketones on positions 3, 6, 11, 17 and 20. While the hydroxyl groups often possess the β configuration, 3α-,

6α-, 17α- and 20α-hydroxyl groups are not uncommon. Hydroxylases which utilize steroids as substrates are also indigenous to the liver. For the most part these enzymes employ cytochrome P_{450} and are microsomal in origin. Predominantly the steroids (neutral or phenolic) are hydroxylated on positions 2, 6, 7, 15 and 16 (28-33).

These hepatic metabolites may be conjugated to glucuronic acid and/or sulfate (or glucosamine) (29). The glucosiduronates re-enter the plasma and are preferentially eliminated through the kidney. The sulfates enter the plasma (see below) or may be eliminated through the bile. One of the characteristics of certain steroids in the enterohepatic circulation is their mixed conjugation with glucuronic acid and sulfate (34).

This hepatic metabolism may positively influence steroid target tissues or hormone dependent neoplasms if it can be assumed that liver steroid metabolites re-enter the circulation. Pharmacological (35) and physiological (36) levels of labeled 17β-estradiol when administered intravenously to pre- and post-menopausal patients have been found in the plasma substantially conjugated to sulfate. After two hours, the fate of the labeled estrogen can be assumed to be the same as that of the endogenous pool of plasma free 17β-estradiol. At this time as much as 2% of the estrogen injected at a physiological level was found in the plasma sulfates. This significant sulfation of plasma free 17β-estradiol probably occurred in the liver. Isolation of 2-methoxyestrone-3-sulfate from the plasma (36) substantiates this premise, since 2-methoxylation of estrogens has been shown to occur only in the liver of non-pregnant women. Investigations from this laboratory (29) and others (37) have demonstrated hepatic 3-sulfation of the estrogen to occur before the 2-position is hydroxylated and the 3-sulfate influences the formation of the 2-methoxy derivative.

At the present time it appears that the estrogens (estrone and 17β-estradiol) are found in the ovaries in the free and 3-sulfate ester form (38). In fact, most of the estrogens in the ovarian venous blood have been isolated as sulfates (10). Once in the plasma, the conjugated, oxidized or reduced state of these estrogens would be expected to be the result of metabolic equilibria between various peripheral tissues, particularly hepatic tissue. In women the conjugated state of administered estrogens isolated from the plasma varied with the subject's age (36). There was a dramatic decrease in the relative quantity of plasma free estrogens which were converted to sulfates as the age of the patient increased. This change was noted just prior to menopause, suggesting that there were alterations in the conjugation of plasma estrogens which were detectable before clinical menopause. At the present time the importance of plasma estrogen sulfates and the relationship of their decrease to the occurrence of menopause is not understood. However, data has been obtained which indicate that in *in vitro* experiments the sulfated estrogens facilitate the uptake of estrogens into rat uterine tissue (17). In addition, estrogen sulfates have been shown to persist in the plasma for a greater period of time than the free estrogens (39).

RELATIONSHIP OF EXCRETED PATTERNS OF STEROID METABOLITES TO BREAST CANCER

Androgens

In their classic studies published over a decade ago, Bulbrook and his co-workers demonstrated empirically that decreased urinary androgen (etiocholanolone) in post-menopausal breast cancer patients accompanied a low remission rate following adrenalectomy or hypophysectomy (40,41). Initially the etiocholanolone levels in the various patients' urines were related utilizing the formula:

$$X = 80-80 \text{ (mg urinary 17}\alpha\text{-hydroxycorticosteroid per 24 hour)} + (\mu\text{g etiocholanolone per 24 hour})$$

where a negative "X" predicted a poor response to hormone ablation (adrenalectomy) and a positive "X" would forecast remission of the tumor following this treatment (42). Remission rates in breast cancer patients correlated well with these discriminants. The decreased androgen excretion in the poor prognosis group of women with breast cancer was attributed to a disorder of adrenocortical function, wherein common precursors of adrenal corticoids and adrenal androgens were diverted from the androgen pathway to the corticoid pathway (43). More recently Zumoff et al (44), utilizing labeled androgen precursors, have demonstrated that the decreased conversion of androgens to urinary 17-ketosteroids was a nonspecific consequence of illness, i.e. not specific for breast cancer. In fact, these investigators showed that the more seriously ill patients presented with the low urinary androgen metabolites and therefore had the poorest prognosis. In regard to the Bulbrook formula these patients would also be most likely to show higher corticoid excretion resulting from their stressed condition and therefore probably a negative discriminant. Lowered urinary levels of 17-ketosteroids have been observed in patients with a wide variety of human diseases (rheumatoid arthritis (45), diabetes mellitis (46), various other cancers (47), cirrhosis (48) and schizophrenia (49)).

Adams and Salasoo (50) demonstrated an intriguing correlation between the increased level (relative to controls) of 16α-hydroxyandrost-5-enes (androst-5-ene-3β,16α-diol-17-one and androst-5-ene-3β,16α,17β-triol) in the urine of patients (breast cancer and other) following operative stress. It was evident in these studies that the 16α-hydroxyandrost-5-enes were excreted at the expense of (or metabolized from) the 17-ketosteroids which had decreased in these urines. This premise was substantiated when a linear relationship was obtained in a plot of urinary 17α-hydroxycorticosteroids versus the sum of the 17-ketosteroids and 16α-hydroxyandrost-5-enes. Furthermore, an earlier report of Adams and Wong (51) showed an increase in urinary androst-5-ene-3β,16α,17β-triol was also accompanied by a decrease in 17-ketosteroids in preoperative (stressed) breast cancer.

It would appear that a decrease in urinary 17-ketosteroids is not as significant in breast cancer or disease as the induced or stimulated conversion of 17-ketosteroids to 16α-hydroxyandrost-5-enes. What then is the relationship between 16α-hydroxylation of steroids and the circumstances of disease?

In experimental animals hepatic mixed oxidases (cytochrome P_{450}) are known to be involved in steroid hydroxlations (52). These microsomal enzymes are responsible for the hydroxylation of steroids at positions 2, 6β, 7β, 15α, 16α, 17α and 21 (28-33,53,54). Other substrates such as fatty acids, drugs, anesthetics, insecticides, and carcinogens are also hydroxylated or oxidatively N-demethylated by this system in the presence of NADPH and oxygen. Both androgens and corticosteroids have been shown to activate this hepatic microsomal mono-oxygenase system although through different mechanisms (55). Apparently androgens increase the binding capacity of substrates to the cytochrome P_{450} while corticosteroids increase the activity of the P_{450} linked NADPH-cytochrome reductase. Estrogens have demonstrated little or no effect on this microsomal enzyme system. More importantly these enzymes are highly inducible and increases in their activities have been observed to approach 10 times following the administration of drugs such as phenobarbital (56). The inducibility of certain cytochrome P_{450} linked enzymes has been demonstrated to be a simple autosomal dominant trait in the mouse (57,58). Various substrates will induce similar or, more often, different hydroxylating activities of hepatic microsomes (55,59). While nearly all of these investigations have been of necessity limited to laboratory animals, a similar induction of the microsomal mixed oxidase has been reported in human leukocytes (60).

Haugen et al have recently recently separated the multiple forms of rabbit hepatic microsomal cytochrome P_{450} (61). Their work revealed the information that the same form of cytochrome P_{450} (P_{450LM_2}) which was induced by phenobarbital administration also formed the 16α-hydroxy androgens. Furthermore, cytochrome P_{450} actively hydroxylated ethyl morphine, a reaction previously demonstrated to increase in the liver of rats exposed to stress or corticosteroids (55).

Based on these investigations with laboratory animals it is reasonable to assume that in breast cancer patients the observed increase in urinary 16α-hydroxy androgens may be directly related to stress and/or the drug regimen of certain patients. Further study of human patients carried out under strictly controlled stress circumstances and drug administration will be necessary to gain greater support for this premise.

In an investigation of the urinary steroids in Guernsey women, Bulbrook and his colleagues have been able to acquire data in a prospective study set up to test the hypothesis that the decrease in 17-ketosteroid excretion preceded the clinical appearance of breast cancer (62). Urine specimens were collected from some 5,000 healthy women. When breast cancer was subsequently discovered in a woman, her prediagnosis excretion of 17-ketosteroids and 17α-hydroxycorticosteroids was compared with matched controls. At the time of publication 27 women had presented with breast cancer. The mean excretion of etiocholanolone in the precancer cases was significantly lower than that of the matched controls. This abnormality in 17-ketosteroids excretion was found at all ages and was seen as early as nine years prior to the diagnosis of breast cancer. The mean time between the collection of urine and subsequent diagnosis was 44 months. Furthermore, these women did not show a difference in their excretion of 17α-hydroxycorticosteroids. The rate of breast cancer incidence was also inversely related to the urinary etiocholanolone urinary level.

The consistency of the urinary level of 17α-hydroxycorticosteroids in patients and controls in this study (62) together with the life style on the Isle of Guernsey would certainly eliminate stress as a contributing factor to the low urinary etiocholanolone and androsterone. *However, considering the above discussion it now appears that the level of the urinary 16α-hydroxyandrost-5-enes in these patients and their matched controls would prove most interesting. Should 16α-hydroxylation of the androgens be established as a cause of low urinary androgens in women prior to the diagnosis of breast cancer, then a much stronger case could be constructed for the involvement of abnormal steroid metabolism in the etiology of breast cancer. Is it possible that these 27 women have higher levels of hepatic mixed oxidase activity specific for 16α-hydroxylation of androgens (i.e. cytochrome $P450_{LM2}$)? How could this metabolic aberration occur? Were the 27 women eventually diagnosed with breast cancer exposed to an unusual drug, pollutant, or dietary regimen consisting of specific inducers of these mixed oxidases? Or could it be that the hepatic cytochrome $P450_{LM2}$ enzymes in the susceptible women are slightly more inducible for genetic reasons? Unfortunately none of these questions can be answered until urinary markers for the various hepatic mixed oxidase activities have been determined in a prospective breast cancer study of women maintained under strictly controlled circumstances.*

Estrogens

Interest in the metabolism of estrogens in breast cancer has prevailed for several decades. Stimulated by the obvious relationship between the estrogens and mammary gland growth and function, numerous laboratories have reported studies of the urinary estrogens in breast cancer patients. With the exception of a few, most of these investigations have been concerned with the three classical estrogens: estrone, 17β-estradiol and estriol. Other estrogen metabolites were simply too difficult to isolate or existed in minute quantities which could not be determined by existing techniques. Initial data from these experiments described both increased estriol excretion(63-65) and decreased estriol excretion (66-68) by breast cancer patients. These conflicting reports have been resolved by the excellent studies of Hellman et al (69) in which the double-isotope-derivative analysis of urinary estrogens was employed. Their data left little doubt that there is an increased peripheral metabolism of endogenous or exogenous estrogens to estriol in breast cancer patients. At the same time there was a normal urinary excretion of estrone, 17β-estradiol, 2-hydroxyestrone, 2-methoxyestrone, and epiestriol. Male breast cancer patients also excreted elevated levels of estriol (70).

Some breast tumors have been shown to contain 16α-hydroxylation capacity when the substrate was dehydroepiandrosterone (71). In addition the A-ring aromatization of the 16α-hydroxylated androgens has been demonstrated in breast tumors by Adams and Wong (72). However, other laboratories have detected only estrone or 17β-estradiol synthesis by certain breast tumors (73,74). This activity was very low and occurred in a minority of tumors. The possible paraendocrine activity of breast tumors would not be expected, therefore, to contribute the relatively large quantities of estriol found in the urine of patients, particularly following the removal of the neoplasm (71). Although estriol secretion by the ovary has been suggested by Longcope et al (75) most of the urinary level of this tri-hydroxy estrogen is formed in the liver of non-pregnant women via 16α-hydroxylation of estrone.

Interestingly, the increased hepatic 16α-hydroxylation of estrogens corresponds with the established induction of 16α-hydroxylation of androgens discussed above and shown to be a nonspecific consequence of illness. Zumoff et al were careful to demonstrate that the increased 16α-hydroxylation of the 17β-estradiol injected into male breast cancer patients was specific to this disease (70). However, the disease specificity of high urinary estriol in female breast cancer patients has not been established. The urine from both the male and female breast cancer patients contained either normal or lower than normal levels of 2-hydroxyestrone and estrone.

The present state of knowledge of steroid metabolism in breast cancer makes it imperative that the possible relationship between the 16α-hydroxylation of androgens and estrogens be further examined. Does the same cytochrome P_{450} linked enzyme (cytochrome $P450_{LM2}$) add hydroxyl groups to the D-ring of both androgens and estrogens? If this were the case, then the coincidence of an increased urinary excretion of 16α-hydroxy androst-5-enes and estriol in patients with breast tumors would be understood. The inability of rat liver to form estriol from estrone (29) while this tissue does contain the necessary enzymes to form 16α-hydroxy-androgens (76) suggests that different enzymatic constituents are required for these two pathways.

In precancerous women considerable data has been accumulated by MacMahon (1,77-79) and Lemon (2,66,80) which indicates a different estrogen metabolic pattern exists before the appearance of the breast tumor. These investigators have utilized the urinary estriol ratio (E_3/E_1+E_2) as a method for equalizing between group variations in estrogen secretion and at the same time giving some information regarding the estrogenicity of the metabolic pattern. Women whose urine contained a low estriol ratio, particularly in the decade following puberty, were shown to have high breast cancer risk (77-79). Furthermore, a survey of the urinary estriol ratios in pre- and post-menopausal women (80) did not yield an average distribution of excretion ratios among the population. Instead Lemon's data (which was plotted utilizing an expanded ordinate capable of resolving 30 or more ratios) showed a polymodal distribution of urinary estriol ratios suggesting several genotypes which were apparently expressed in the degree of 16α-hydroxylation of estrogens.

Therefore, it would appear that low estriol formation is characteristic of estrogen metabolism prior to the disease. However, examination of the data* (81) reveals that urinary estriol levels are not different between high and low risk populations. Instead the low risk breast cancer group excreted decreased levels of estrone and 17β-estradiol. Several groups of investigators have interpreted these results as an indication that the higher relative level of weakly estrogenic compounds (e.g. estriol) "protects" target tissues from the carcinogenic (77,81) effect of the more active estrogens. Since pregnancy results in very high levels of urinary estriol, this viewpoint has been extrapolated to explain the protecting effect of early first pregnancy on the incidence of breast

*During the preparation of this manuscript an excellent review entitled "Hormone Profiles in Hormone-Dependent Cancers" by B. Zumoff et al was published in Cancer Research (81). Although this publication did not appear in time to be included in the Symposium round table discussions (Steroid Hormone Action and Cancer), I am grateful for the opportunity to incorporate into this manuscript certain concepts of these authors.

cancer (78). In line with this reasoning, the "anti-estrogenic" activity of estriol has been mentioned as an inhibitor of the carcinogenic process, particularly since estriol competes with 17β-estradiol at the level of receptor binding in target tissues (80). However, it must be stated at this point that estriol has been shown not only to be anti-carcinogenic (82) but, conversely, to produced mammary tumors in rodents (where this estrogen does not normally exist, 83). Furthermore, the levels of free estriol (i.e. not conjugated to glucouronic acid) in the plasma which is in contact with the tissues is naturally very low and in no way related to the estriol glucosiduronate which is excreted. Regarding the "pulse" of estriol in pregnancy being protective during the decade or more required for the carcinogenic process, this is very difficult to visualize in the light of present understanding of the receptor mechanism of steroid hormone activity in target tissues which does not predict a long residence of the steroid within the cell or nucleus. Nor does the theory predict passage of the nuclear bound steroid nor its influence to daughter cells.

A recent report from the laboratories of Jack Fishman has indicated that one of the major plasma estrogens in women is 2-hydroxyestrone (84). This labile metabolite, previously lost in most assay procedures, was shown through radioimmunoassay to exist in the plasma in concentrations equal to that of estrone plus 17β-estradiol. 2-Hydroxyestrone would be a better anti-estrogen in "protecting" target tissues from the carcinogenic process (81) since this compound exists free in the plasma and is a better competitor for the estrogen receptor than estriol (81,85). Therefore, according to Zumoff et al (81) "normal" plasma levels of this metabolite may conceivably continually protect target tissues from the postulated carcinogenic potential of more active estrogens.

All of the previous work relating breast cancer to urinary estrogens must now be re-evaluated in the light of this elusive but important metabolite. For example, the "estriol ratio" would obviously increase with the increased conversion of estrone to 2-hydroxyestrone. Hellman et al (69) demonstrated in female breast cancer patients that the urinary 2-hydroxy estrogen did not change appreciably while estriol did increase. However, is decreased hepatic synthesis of 2-hydroxyestrone characteristic of breast cancer prone women? While this estrogen has been found in urine, nothing is known regarding its formation in relation to the production of estriol. Both metabolites are assumed to be synthesized on the hepatic microsomes (for the most part) via the cytochrome P_{450} system. To this end, it would be important to know the relationship between the hepatic mixed oxidase system specific for the 16α-hydroxylation of estrogens and androgens and that system specific for the 2-hydroxylation of estrogens.

THE POSITIVE INFLUENCE OF HEPATIC TISSUE IN STEROID HORMONE HOMEOSTASIS

Classical endocrinology has long viewed the liver as an organ important only in the elimination of steroid hormones and their precursors. This discussion of steroid metabolism in breast cancer has assigned hepatic tissue a more influential role in steroid hormone homeostasis and target tissue control than previously imagined. Some very recent observations suggest such an effective function for the liver.

In recent years it became apparent that the hepatic steroid metabolic patterns were different in males and females (86). It was not until the investigations of Gustafsson and DeMoor that some light was shed on this phenomenon (27,28,30-33). The female pattern of hepatic steroid metabolism was observed to continue from birth until puberty in both sexes, at which time the male livers began to form predominantly the 5β-reduced C_{19} steroid containing hydroxyls at positions 2α and β, 3α, 6β, 16α. On the other hand, both the female juvenile and adult patterns contained as the major C_{19} steroid metabolites the 5α-reduced, 3α- and 7α-hydroxlated steroids. Liver tissue from the male rat would continue to metabolize steroids in the female pattern if the animal was castrated during the first ten days after birth. From these studies it became clear that the metabolic fate of steroids in the liver was determined during the neonatal period.

Gustafsson et al (87) have proceeded to show that the female pattern of steroid metabolism was brought about by neonatal exposure of hepatic tissue to the follicle stimulating hormone. Interestingly, Dohler and Wuttle have reported that, in the neonatal female plasma, FSH reached extremely high levels, while in the male the endogenous neonatal androgens block the pituitary secretion of these high FSH levels (88). Direct evidence that these hepatic steroid metabolites possess peripheral activities which are manifested in masculinity or feminity is still lacking. However, observations of neonatally castrated male rats have revealed decreased aggressiveness and a lessened mounting instinct (89). It follows then, that the liver is a metabolically responsive target tissue for certain pituitary hormones, and furthermore, this tissue through its metabolism of steroids may positively influence target tissues.

CONCLUSION

In retrospect, the long fascinating relationship between breast cancer and urinary steroid patterns can be attributed to variations in hepatic steroid metabolism. These metabolic variants are now known to be representative of the highly inducible microsomal oxidase systems (cytochrome P_{450}), the inducibility of which has been demonstrated in rodents to be genetically determined. To date, the inducers for these systems have been shown to include foreign compounds such as certain drugs and environmental pollutents or carcinogens. The activity of these hepatic mixed oxidases may also be stimulated by the corticosteroids resulting from stress.

The challenge to those dedicated to the study of breast cancer resides in the establishment of whether these unusual quantitative differences in steroid hormone metabolism are directly responsible for the carcinogenic process in the breast; or do these metabolic aberrations simply serve to indicate a general alteration of the body's functions which, through other routes, results in breast cancer?

REFERENCES

1. MacMahon, B. and P. Cole, Cancer 24:1146, 1969.

2. Lemon, H.M., Cancer 25:423, 1970.

3. Smith, O.W. and G.V. Smith, The Lancet I: 1152, 1970.

4. Wynder, E.L., Cancer 24:1235, 1969.

5. Dao, T.L., In: Wissler, R.W., T.L. Dao and S. Wood (eds.), Endogenous Factors Influencing Host-Tumor Balance, University of Chicago Press, Chicago, 1967, p. 75.

6. Stocks, P., Brit. J. Cancer 24:633, 1970.

7. Hems, G., Brit. J. Cancer 24:226, 1970.

8. Bulbrook, R.D., J.L. Haywood and C.C. Spicer, The Lancet II, 395, 1971.

9. Gardner, W.U., Cancer 17:1092, 1958.

10. Giorgi, E.P., J. Endocrinol. 37:211, 1967.

11. Sneddon, A. and G.F. Marrian, Biochem. J. 86:385, 1963.

12. Hudson, B. and G.W. Ortel, Anal. Biochem. 2:248, 1961.

13. Gallegos, A.J. and D.L. Berliner, J. Clin. Endocrinol. 27: 1214, 1967.

14. Kim, M.H. and W.L. Herrmann, J. Clin. Endocrinol. 28:187, 1968.

15. Mainwaring, W.I.P., Biochim. Biophys. Res. Comm. 49:192, 1970.

16. Thieulant, M.-L., L. Mercier, S. Samperez, P. Jouan, J. Steroid Biochem. 6:1257, 1975.

17. Pack, B.A. and S.C. Brooks, Endocrinology 87:924, 1970.

18. Tseng, L. and E. Gurpide, Endocrinology 94:419, 1974.

19. Makman, M.H., S. Nakagawa and A. White, Rec. Prog. Horm. Res. 24:195, 1967.

20. Pack, B.A. and S.C. Brooks, Endocrinology 95:1680, 1974.

21. Bolt, W., F. Rital and H.M. Bolt, Verh. dtsch. Ges. inn. Med. 71:461, 1966.

22. Schindler, A.E., A. Ebert and E. Friedrich, J. Clin. Endocrinol. 35:627, 1972.

23. Longcope, C., T. Kato and R. Horton, J. Clin. Invest. 48: 2191, 1969.

24. Zumoff, B., J. Fishman, T.F. Gallagher and L. Hellman, J. Clin. Invest. 47:20, 1968.

25. Adlercreutz, H., J. Endocrinol. 46:129, 1970.

26. Plaa, G.L. and R.E. Larson, Arch. Environ. Health 9:536, 1964.

27. DeMoor, P., G. Verhoeven and W. Heyns, Differentiation 1: 241, 1973.

28. Gustafsson, J.-A., S.A. Gustafsson, Eur. J. Biochem. 44:225, 1974.

29. Brooks, S.C. and L. Horn, Biochim. Biophys. Acta 231:233, 1971.

30. Gustafsson, J.-A., A. Stenberg, J. Biol. Chem. 249:711, 1974.

31. Gustafsson, J.-A., A. Stenberg, J. Biol. Chem. 249:719, 1974.

32. Berg, A. and J.-A. Gustafsson, J. Biol. Chem. 248:6559, 1973.

33. Gustafsson, J.-A. and M. Ingelman-Sundberg, J. Biol. Chem. 249:1940, 1974.

34. Aldercreutz, H. and T. Luukkainen, Acta Endocr. Suppl. 124: 101, 1967.

35. Purdy, R.H., L.L. Engel and J.L. Oncley, J. Biol. Chem. 236: 1043, 1961.

36. Vaughn, C.B., D. Kolakowski, V. Zylka and S.C. Brooks, J. Clin. Endocrinol., Submitted for publication.

37. Miyazaki, M., I. Yoshizawa and J. Fishman, Biochem. 8:1669, 1969.

38. Wallace, E. and N. Silberman, J. Biol. Chem. 239:2809, 1964.

39. Ruder, H.J., D.L. Loriaux and M.B. Lipsett, J. Clin. Invest. 51:1020, 1972.

40. Bulbrook, R.D., J.L. Hayward, C.C. Spicer and B.S. Thomas, Lancet II: 1235, 1962.

41. Bulbrook, R.D., J.L. Hayward, C.C. Spicer and B.S. Thomas, Lancet II: 1238, 1962.

42. Bulbrook, R.D., F.C. Greenwood and J.L. Hayward, Lancet II: 1154, 1960.

43. Deshpande, N., V. Jensen, R.D. Bulbrook and T.W. Douss, Steroids 9:393, 1967.

44. Zumoff, B., H.L. Bradlow, T.F. Gallagher and L. Hellman, J. Clin. Endocrinol. 32:824, 1971.

45. Davison, R.A., P. Koets and W.C. Kuzell, J. Clin. Endocrinol. 7:201, 1947.

46. Miller, S. and H.L. Mason, J. Clin. Endocrinol. 5:220, 1945.

47. Rhoads, C.P., K. Dobriner, E. Gordan, L.F. Fieser and S. Lieberman, Trans. Assoc. Amer. Physicians 57:203, 1942.

48. Lloyd, C.W. and R.H. Williams, Amer. J. Med. 4:315, 1948.

49. Gottfried, S.P. and I. Minsky, AMA Arch. Neurol. Physch. 66: 708, 1951.

50. Adams, J.B. and S. Salasoo, Acta Endocrinol. 72:319, 1973.

51. Adams, J.B. and M.S.F. Wong, Lancet II: 1163, 1968.

52. Kupfer, D. and S. Orrenius, Eur. J. Biochem. 14:317, 1970.

53. Hrycay, E.G. and P.J. O'Brien, Arch. Biochem. Biophys. 153: 480, 1972.

54. Cooper, D.Y., S. Narasimhulu, O. Rosenthal and R.W. Estabrook, In: McKerns, K.W. (ed.), Functions of the Adrenal Cortex, Vol. II, Appleton-Century-Crofts, Inc., New York, 1968, p. 897.

55. Hamrik, M.E., N.G. Zampaglione, B. Stripp and J.R. Gillette, Biochem. Pharm. 22:293, 1973.

56. Leven, W.R., M. Welch and A.H. Conney, Endocrinology 80:135, 1967.

57. Nebert, D.W., E.M. Goujon and J.E. Gielen, Nature New Biol. 236:107, 1972.

58. Robinson, J.P., N. Considine and D.W. Nebert, J. Biol. Chem. 249:5851, 1974.

59. Lu, A.Y.H. and W. Leven, Biochem. Biophys. Res. Comm. 46: 1334, 1972.

60. Kellermann, G., E. Cantrell and C.R. Shaw, Cancer Res. 33: 1654, 1973.

61. Haugen, D.A., T.A. Van der Hoeven and M.J. Coon, J. Biol. Chem. 250:3567, 1975.

62. Bulbrook, R.D., J.L. Hayward and C.C. Spicer, Lancet, 395, 1971.

63. Persson, B.H. and L. Risholm, Acta Endocrinol. 47:15, 1964.

64. Marmorsten, J., L.G. Crowley, S.M. Myers, E. Stern and C.E. Hopkins, Amer. J. Obstet. Gynec. 92:462, 1965.

65. Nissen-Meyer, R. and T. Sanner, Acta Endocrinol. 44:334, 1963.

66. Lemon, H.M., H.H. Wotiz, L. Parsons and P.J. Mozden, JAMA 196: 1128, 1966.

67. Bacigalupo, G. and K. Schubert, Klin. Wschr. 38:804, 1960.

68. Schweppe, J.S., R.A. Jungman and I. Lewis, Cancer 20:155, 1967.

69. Hellman, L., B. Zumoff, J. Fishman and T.F. Gallagher, J. Clin. Endocrinol. 33:138, 1971.

70. Zumoff, B., J. Fishman, J. Cassouto, L. Hellman and T.F. Gallagher, J. Clin. Endocrinol. 26:960, 1966.

71. Adams, J.B. and M.S.F. Wong, J. Endocrinol. 41:41, 1968.

72. Adams, J.B. and M.S.F. Wong, In: Dao T.L. (ed.), Estrogens, Target Tissues and Neoplasia, University of Chicago Press, Chicago, 1972, p. 125.

73. Dao, T.L., R. Varela and C. Morreal, In: Dao, T.L. (ed.), Estrogens, Target Tissues and Neoplasia, University of Chicago Press, Chicago, 1972, p. 163.

74. Abul-Hajj, Y.J., Steroids 26:488, 1975.

75. Rotti, K., J. Stevens, D. Watson and C. Longcope, Steroids 25:807, 1975.

76. Lu, A.Y.H., R. Kuntzman, S. West, M. Jacobson and A.H. Conney, J. Biol. Chem. 247:1727, 1972.

77. Cole, P. and B. MacMahon, Lancet I:604, 1969.

78. MacMahon, B. and P. Cole, J. Natl. Can. Inst. 50:21, 1973.

79. MacMahon, B., P. Cole, J.B. Brown, K. Aoki, T.M. Lin, R.W. Morgan and N.C. Woo, Intern. J. Cancer 14:161, 1974.

80. Lemon, H.M., J. Surg. Oncol. 4:255, 1972.

81. Zumoff, B., J. Fishman, H.L. Bradley and L. Hellman, Cancer Res. 35:3365, 1975.

82. Lemon, H.M., Cancer Res. 13:1341, 1975.

83. Rudali, G., F. Apiou and B. Muel, Eur. J. Cancer 4:39, 1975.

84. Yoshizawa, I. and J. Fishman, J. Clin. Endocrinol. 32:3, 1971.

85. Davies, I.J., F. Naftolin, K.J. Ryan, J. Fishman and J. Siu, Endocrinology 97:554, 1975.

86. Einarsson, K., J.-A. Gustafsson and A.J. Goldman, Eur. J. Biochem. 31:345, 1972.

87. Gustafsson, J.-A. and A. Stenberg, Endocrinology 96:501, 1975.

88. Dohler, K.D. and W. Wuttke, Endocrinology 94:1003, 1974.

89. Davidson, J.M. and S. Levine, Ann. Rev. Physiol. 34:375, 1972.

FRACTIONATION OF DIVERSE STEROID-BINDING PROTEINS: BASIC AND CLINICAL APPLICATIONS

Merry R. Sherman and Lorraine K. Miller

Memorial Sloan-Kettering Cancer Center

New York, New York 10021

Two types of diversity in steroid-binding proteins have become apparent: 1) the presence of several intracellular receptors and/or serum steroid-binding components in a tissue; and 2) the existence of multiple forms of individual receptors. Resolution of these components is clearly essential to understanding the mechanisms of action of one or more steroids in a target cell. The techniques that can be used to fractionate such mixtures and characterize the constituents include analytical gel filtration, polyacrylamide gel electrophoresis, preparative ion exchange filtration and polyamine precipitation, in addition to density gradient centrifugation. Applications of these techniques to a clinical problem, the influence of steroids on breast cancer, and a fundamental problem, the subunit structure of chick oviduct progesterone receptors, will be described in this chapter.

PREPARATION OF TISSUES FOR ANALYSIS

All procedures were carried out at 0 to 4 C. Breast specimens or chick oviducts were homogenized in 5 ml/g of 10mM N-tris(hydroxymethyl)methyl-2-aminoethanesulfonic acid (Tes)*, 12mM thioglycerol,

---

*Abbreviations used are: Bis, N,N'-methylenebisacrylamide; DEAE, diethylaminoethyl; DES, diethylstilbestrol; DHT or dihydrotestosterone, 5α-dihydrotestosterone; E_2 or estradiol, 17β-estradiol; E_1, estrone; HSA, human serum albumin; SBG, sex steroid binding globulin (testosterone-estradiol binding globulin); Tes, N-tris(hydroxymethyl)methyl-2-aminoethanesulfonic acid; Tes-thioglycerol, 10mM Tes, 12mM thioglycerol, pH 7.4.

pH 7.4 (Tes-thioglycerol), containing 0.25 M sucrose. The high speed supernatant fraction (cytosol) was prepared by a conventional method (1) and stored at -80 C. Mixtures of ^{3}H-steroids and unlabelled competitors in ethanol were added to thawed cytosol or serum to a maximum ethanol concentration of 3% v/v.

ESTROGEN-BINDING PROTEINS OF BREAST TUMOR CYTOSOL AND SERUM: ANALYTICAL GEL FILTRATION VS CHARCOAL-DEXTRAN ASSAYS

Gel filtration was performed on columns of Agarose A-0.5m (23 x 1.27 cm) in Tes-thioglycerol containing 0.4 M KCl and 10% w/v glycerol. Duplicate columns were mounted on opposite sides of an LKB fraction collector (UltroRac) so that samples labelled with ^{3}H-steroid $\pm$ a competitor or with two different competitors could be analyzed simultaneously. The elution volumes of proteins such as myoglobin, serum albumin and ovalbumin were monitored optically as standards for the calculation of the molecular radii of the steroid binding components (2).

Gel filtration patterns of human breast tumor cytosol and serum labelled with ^{3}H-estradiol $\pm$ various competitors are shown in Figs 1 and 2. The free ^{3}H-estradiol (open symbols in Fig 1) was retarded significantly beyond the total liquid volume (V_t) as measured by the elution of ^{14}C-valine. This retardation improved the resolution of bound from free steroid, but indicated the presence of interactions between the steroid and the gel that may decrease the binding detected by this technique. In this high salt buffer, the complex formed by ^{3}H-estradiol and breast tumor cytosol was eluted just after albumin. The radioactivity associated with this component was virtually eliminated by 100-fold excesses of either unlabelled estradiol or diethylstilbestrol. Lower ratios of unlabelled competitor to labelled steroid (e.g., 10:1, 1:1, 0.1:1) would be required to distinguish between the affinities for the natural and synthetic compounds. The affinity of estrone was intermediate between those of estradiol and dihydrotestosterone; the latter caused no detectable decrease in ^{3}H-estradiol binding at a molar ratio of 100:1.

While our current protocol includes a request for serum with every tumor specimen, serum was not available from the patient whose cytosol was analyzed in Fig 1. Therefore, analogous studies are illustrated for the serum from a normal premenopausal woman (Fig 2). There were several important differences between the results obtained with the normal serum and the tumor cytosol. The apparent ratio of bound to free steroid in undiluted serum was much higher than in cytosol incubated with the same ^{3}H-estradiol concentration (2×10^{-8}M). This difference reflects the higher binding capacity of the serum protein(s) and implies that a small amount of

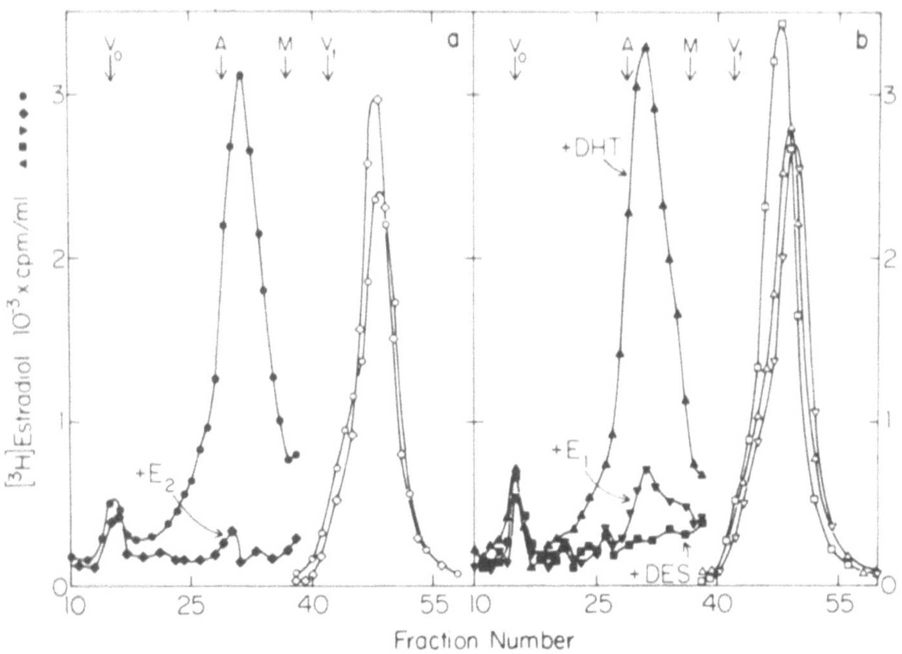

Fig 1. Agarose Gel Filtration of Human Breast Tumor Estrogen Receptors. Tumor cytosol from a postmenopausal woman was incubated for 4 hrs at 4 C with 2 x 10^{-8}M ^{3}H-estradiol $\pm$ 2 x 10^{-6}M unlabelled estradiol (E_2), estrone (E_1), dihydrotestosterone (DHT) or diethylstilbestrol (DES). Aliquots (125µl) were filtered on 30ml columns of Agarose A-0.5m (BioRad) in 0.4 M KCl, 10% w/v glycerol in Tes-thioglycerol. The elution volumes of human serum albumin (A), myoglobin (M) and ^{14}C-valine, a marker of the total liquid volume (V_t), are indicated. The void volume (V_o) was measured with Blue Dextran in the absence of cytosol. The labelled complex was eluted just after albumin and had relative affinities DES $\approx$ E_2 > E_1 > DHT.

contaminating serum could account for the quantity of steroid bound by the cytosol. The serum and cytosol complexes were distinguishable, however, both by their molecular radii and by their binding specificities. The serum complex was eluted slightly ahead of albumin under these conditions, and had relative affinities of dihydrotestosterone > estradiol > estrone > diethylstilbestrol. These properties are characteristic of sex steroid binding globulin (SBG) (3,4).

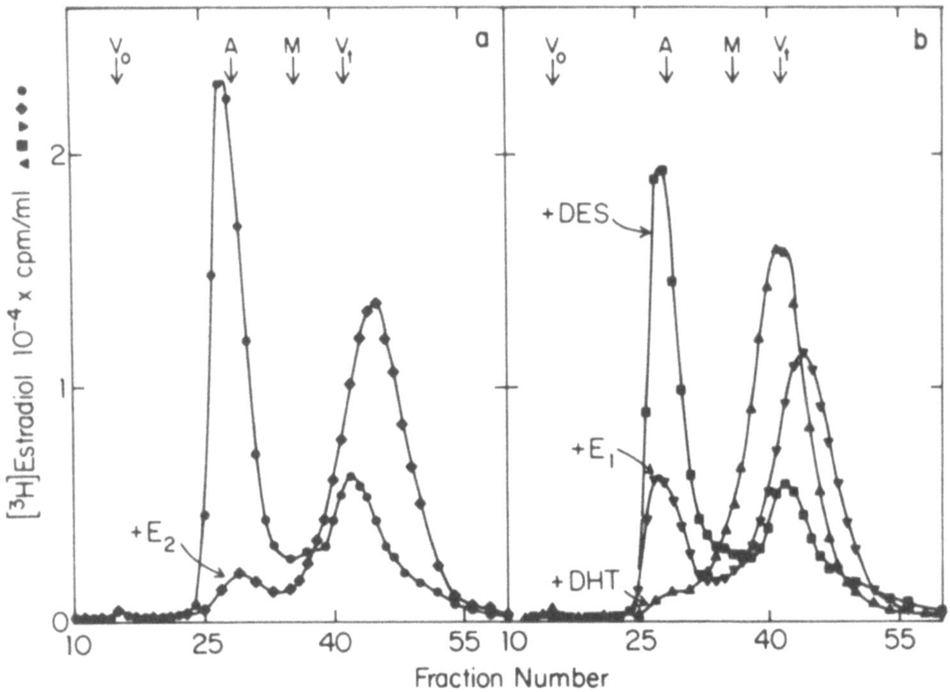

Fig 2. Gel Filtration of Premenopausal Serum Labelled with ^{3}H-Estradiol $\pm$ Competitors. Undiluted serum was incubated with steroids and 100μl aliquots were fractionated as in Fig 1. The labelled complex was eluted before albumin (A) and showed relative affinities DHT > E_2 > E_1 > DES.

The preceding gel filtration data were compared with charcoal-dextran assays of similarly labelled samples. As shown in Table I, the charcoal-resistant binding of ^{3}H-estradiol to tumor cytosol from different patients was decreased to a variable extent by dihydrotestosterone. This technique does not discriminate between the possible cross-reaction of the androgen with intracellular estrogen receptors and contamination of the cytosol with a serum protein that binds both sex steroids. The advantages of techniques like gel filtration, that physically separate the binding components, are thus apparent. On the other hand, the poor resolution obtained by gel filtration between two serum proteins known to bind steroids, albumin and SBG (Fig 2), points out the need for fractionation methods based on molecular properties other than size.

TABLE I

Charcoal-Dextran Assay of Competitive Steroid Binding to Breast Tumor Cytosol and Serum from the Same Patient

Patient	J	L1	L2	M	P	S
Breast Tumor Cytosol						
No Competitor	4.6	2.0	3.0	14.3	1.2	1.4
Diethylstilbestrol	1.5	1.0	1.0	1.9	0.6	0.4
Estradiol	1.3	1.0	-	1.9	-	-
Estrone	-	-	-	3.8	-	-
Dihydrotestosterone	4.6	1.2	2.7	10.0	0.7	0.6
Serum						
No Competitor	31.2	22.7	13.5	-	21.8	32.7
Diethylstilbestrol	29.3	22.7	12.0	-	15.2	18.4
Estradiol	13.5	14.0	12.0	-	14.7	10.7
Estrone	-	-	-	-	13.8	-
Dihydrotestosterone	9.3	13.8	6.6	-	10.5	7.7

Cytosol and serum were incubated for 4 hrs at 4 C with 2 x 10^{-8}M ^{3}H-estradiol $\pm$ 2 x 10^{-6}M unlabelled competitors. Aliquots were counted to verify the total ^{3}H-estradiol concentration. One-fourth volume of 2.5% Norit A (acid washed), 0.25% Dextran T-40 in Tes-thioglycerol was added, shaken vigorously for 20 min, centrifuged at 1000 x g for 15 min and an aliquot of the supernatant was counted (16). The results are given as the percentage of the total ^{3}H-estradiol bound (i.e., 100 x charcoal-resistant dpm/total dpm in the sample). Other aliquots of the cytosol of patient M were analyzed by gel filtration (Fig 1).

ELECTROPHORESIS OF SERUM STEROID-BINDING PROTEINS AND STANDARDS

Corvol et al (4) were the first to analyze a serum steroid-binding protein by electrophoresis in polyacrylamide gels of systematically varied concentration. The electrophoretic resolution among multiple steroid-binding proteins in human serum is illustrated in Figs 3 and 4. Electrophoresis was performed as described by Miller et al (5) in a modification of Davis' (6) Tris-glycine-HCl buffer system. The total concentration of acrylamide (T) in the separation gels was varied from 5 to 15% w/v, including the cross-linking agent, N,N'-methylenebisacrylamide (Bis) and the

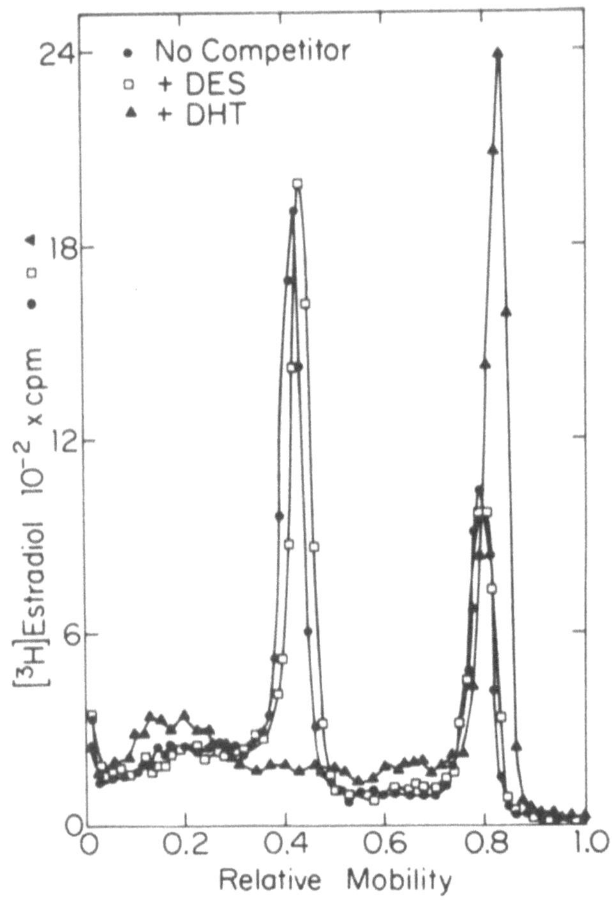

Fig 3. Electrophoretic Assays of Competitive Steroid Binding to Premenopausal Serum. Undiluted serum from the same woman as in Fig 2 was incubated with 2×10^{-8}M ^{3}H-estradiol without a competitor (•) or with a 100-fold excess of unlabelled diethylstilbestrol (DES, □) or dihydrotestosterone (DHT, ▲) for 4 hrs at 4 C. Aliquots (20μl) were electrophoresed on 15% C, 5% T separation gels with 20% C, 3% T stacking gels (5). The labelled complexes with relative mobilities of about 0.4 and 0.8 under these conditions were identified as sex steroid binding globulin (SBG) and serum albumin (HSA), respectively. ^{3}H-Estradiol binding to HSA was increased when unlabelled DHT blocked its binding to SBG. No competition by DES was evident.

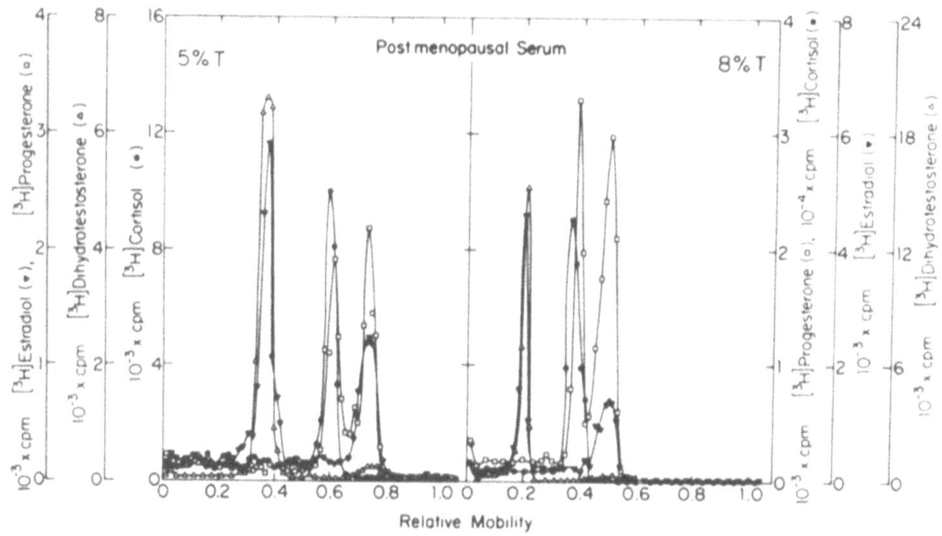

Fig 4. Electrophoretic Resolution of Steroid-Binding Components of Similar Size. Serum from a postmenopausal patient was incubated with 5 x 10^{-9}M ^{3}H-estradiol (E_2), ^{3}H-progesterone (P), ^{3}H-dihydrotestosterone (DHT) or ^{3}H-cortisol (F) for 1 hr at 4 C. Aliquots (40μl) were electrophoresed on separation gels containing 2% C and 5 or 8% T, with 20% C, 3% T stacking gels. The Tris-glycine-HCl buffer system of Davis (6) was supplemented with 10% w/v glycerol. The binding components were identified by their respective specificities: sex steroid-binding globulin, labelled by E_2 and DHT, had the lowest relative mobility (R_f), corticosteroid-binding globulin, labelled by P and F, had intermediate R_f, and serum albumin, labelled by E_2 and P, had the highest R_f.

monomer. In some experiments the porosity of the gels was increased by increasing the ratio of Bis/monomer to 15/85. In other words, the gels were highly cross-linked (15% C) compared to conventional gels (2% C) (7).

Fig 3 shows electrophoretic analyses of human serum labelled with ^{3}H-estradiol in the presence and absence of competing hormones. There are two major differences between these results and the corresponding gel filtration patterns in Fig 2. First, there is clear resolution between albumin, relative mobility (R_f) = 0.8, and sex steroid binding globulin (SBG), R_f = 0.4, despite their similar sizes. Second, significant binding of ^{3}H-estradiol (and ^{3}H-progesterone, see below) to albumin is detectable. This difference in binding observed by the two techniques can be attributed to the intense concentration of the proteins during electrophoretic stacking (with or without a stacking gel) and to the short time required for fractionation (4 hrs in 110 mm separation gels at 2 ma/gel). The rapid dissociation rate constant (and corresponding high equilibrium dissociation constant) of the steroid-albumin interactions preclude their detection by most other techniques (cf. Fig 2).

The results in Fig 3 illustrate an occurrence that may be common in analyses of competitive steroid binding to mixtures of proteins: When excess dihydrotestosterone prevented the binding of ^{3}H-estradiol to the higher affinity, lower capacity sites on SBG, more ^{3}H-estradiol was available to bind to the lower affinity, higher capacity sites on albumin. This type of apparent "shift" of ^{3}H-steroid from a low capacity to a high capacity binding protein could also occur during homogenization of a labelled tumor specimen in the presence of contaminating serum.

Electrophoretic analyses of human serum labelled with four different ^{3}H-steroids (5×10^{-9}M) are shown in Fig 4. Unlike the intracellular steroid receptors (cf. Fig 6), all three steroid-binding proteins of serum migrate well in polyacrylamide gels polymerized with the usual cross-linking (2% C) and a range of total acrylamide concentrations.

The resolution among multiple (steroid-binding) proteins and the information obtained about them is increased dramatically by performing electrophoresis in gels of several concentrations. As first recognized by Ferguson (8) from experiments in starch gels, the contributions of molecular size and net charge to the relative electrophoretic mobility (R_f) can be distinguished by studying log R_f as a function of total gel concentration (T). Chrambach and Rodbard (9) analyzed both theoretically and empirically the application to polyacrylamide gels of the Ferguson plot,

$$\log R_f = \log Y_o - K_R T$$

in which the intercept ($\log Y_o$) is a function primarily of net charge and the negative slope or retardation coefficient (K_R) is a function primarily of molecular size. These relationships have been discussed in detail elsewhere (10,11). It is sufficient to illustrate here the results for a few of the standard proteins studied under the same conditions as the steroid-binding proteins of human serum (Fig 3) and chick oviduct cytosol (Figs 6-8). As shown in Fig 5, the Ferguson plots for two dissimilar proteins, e.g., myoglobin and thyroglobulin or hemoglobin and ferritin, may intersect because of compensating size and charge effects. Thus, if electrophoresis had been performed in this buffer system only in gels of 6% T, neither of these pairs of proteins would have been resolved.

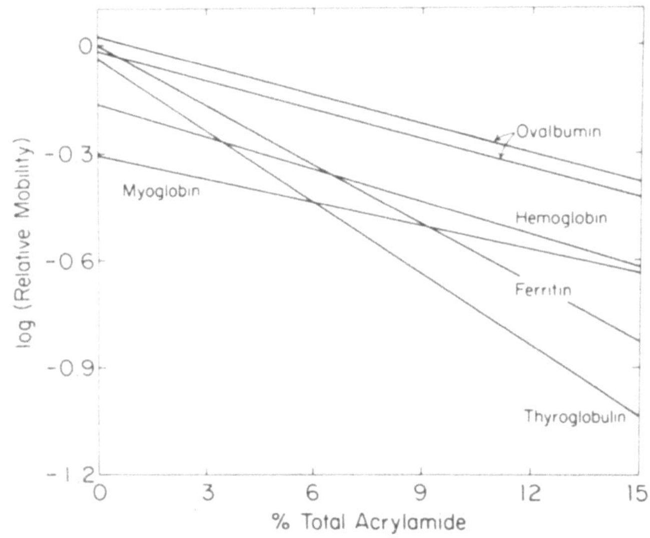

Fig 5. Systematic Electrophoresis of Standard Proteins under the Conditions Used for Receptors. Electrophoresis was performed in 15% C separation gels containing 5, 7, 9, 11, 13 or 15% T, with 20% C, 3% T stacking gels in a Tris-glycine-HCl buffer system (5). Samples containing 15μl of protein (10 mg/ml) in the stacking gel buffer with 20% v/v glycerol were layered over 75μl of 50% glycerol containing 5 μmoles of Tris-thioglycolate, a reducing agent. Following electrophoresis, the gels were dipped in $AgNO_3$ to visualize the chloride-thioglycolate boundary, proteins were stained with Amido Black and the background was destained with acetic acid. Protein mobilities (R_f's) were calculated relative to the chloride-thioglycolate boundary. Weighted linear regressions of log R_f on T (Ferguson plots) were computed with the program of D. Rodbard. Two bands of nearly equal intensity were detected in all analyses of ovalbumin. Data for minor bands in myoglobin and thyroglobulin are not shown.

ELECTROPHORESIS OF INTRACELLULAR RECEPTORS IN HIGHLY CROSS-LINKED POLYACRYLAMIDE GELS

As illustrated in Fig 4, adequate resolution among multiple steroid-binding proteins in serum was obtained by electrophoresis in conventional gels. Analyses of target organ cytosol labelled with ^3H-steroids in such gels, however, were unsatisfactory, since most of the radioactivity remained at the top of the gel. Typical results for chick oviduct progesterone receptors in 2% C gels are shown in Fig 6. The higher mobility cytosol component had an $R_f <$ 0.2 in the 7% T gel and $<$ 0.1 in the 11% T gel. Such results would

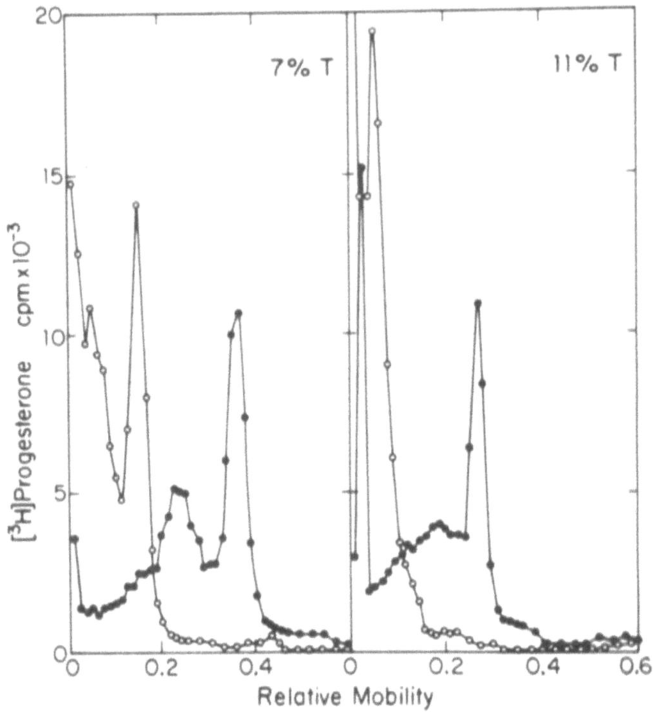

Fig 6. Effect of Cross-Linking on Electrophoretic Mobilities of Chick Oviduct Progesterone Receptors. Oviduct cytosol was incubated with 4 x 10^{-8}M ^{3}H-progesterone for 3 hrs at 4 C. Aliquots (25μl) were electrophoresed as described by Miller et al (5). The relative concentrations (C) of the cross-linking agent N,N'-methylenebisacrylamide (Bis) to the total acrylamide (monomer + Bis) in the 3-ml separation gels were 2% (o) or 15% (•), w/w. The total acrylamide concentrations (T) were 7% (left) or 11% (right), w/v. The 0.5-ml stacking gels contained 20% C and 3% T. (From 5 and unpublished data).

not be suitable for Ferguson plot analysis of size and net charge. The slower cytosol components moved only a short distance in the 7% gels and were completely excluded from the 11% T gels. The improved resolution of both the components in the highly cross-linked (15% C) gels is shown in filled symbols in Fig 6.

The application of highly cross-linked polyacrylamide gels to the fractionation of the subcomponents of the oviduct progesterone receptor is shown in Fig 7. As in an earlier study (1), agarose filtration of oviduct cytosol in the presence of > 0.3 M KCl provided

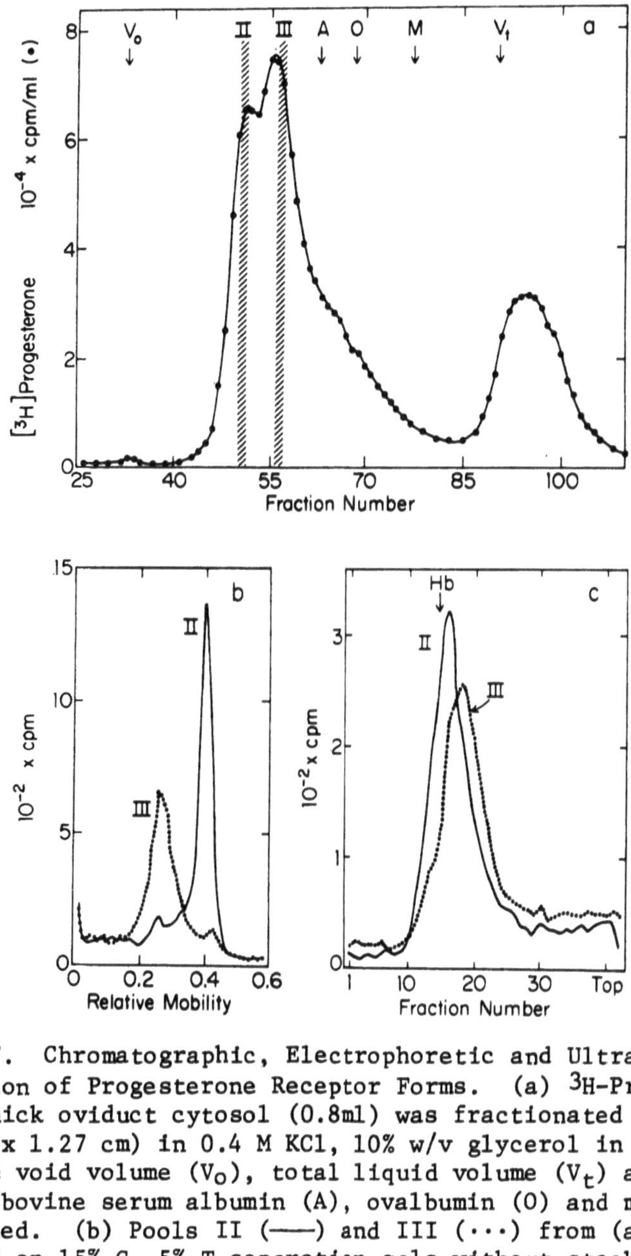

Fig 7. Chromatographic, Electrophoretic and Ultracentrifugal Fractionation of Progesterone Receptor Forms. (a) ^3H-Progesterone-labelled chick oviduct cytosol (0.8ml) was fractionated on Agarose A-0.5m (88 x 1.27 cm) in 0.4 M KCl, 10% w/v glycerol in Tes-thioglycerol. The void volume (V_o), total liquid volume (V_t) and elution volumes of bovine serum albumin (A), ovalbumin (O) and myoglobin (M) are indicated. (b) Pools II (——) and III (···) from (a) were electrophoresed on 15% C, 5% T separation gels without stacking gels, (c) Aliquots (0.2ml) of pools II and III from (a) were centrifuged for 45 hrs at 227,000 x g through 10 to 35% w/v glycerol gradients in a Tris-glycine buffer, pH 10.2, with hemoglobin (Hb) as an internal standard. The mean sedimentation coefficients of forms II and III in four experiments were 4.2 and 3.9 S, respectively. Data from (13).

only partial resolution of two progesterone-binding components (II and III in Fig 7a). When aliquots of the column eluate were electrophoresed in 15% C, 5% T gels, however, the two components were completely separated (Fig 7b). The lack of resolution of the same conponents by density gradient centrifugation in the operative buffer of the electrophoretic system is shown in Fig 7c.

FRACTIONATION OF RECEPTOR FORMS BY ION EXCHANGE FILTRATION AND PROTAMINE PRECIPITATION

Santi et al (12) introduced the use of ion exchange filters to assess the amount of protein-bound steroid. We modified this technique to a small-scale preparative method for the fractionation of mixtures of steroid-binding proteins. Cytosol or serum labelled with ^{3}H-steroid was applied to diethylaminoethyl-(DEAE) cellulose filter paper disks. For example, 0.1 ml of cytosol was placed on each of seven filters (24 mm diameter, Whatman DE-81) on a manifold (Hoefer Model FH 204) connected to a vacuum. After a 1-min adsorption, the vacuum was turned on, the filters were washed with buffer to remove unbound steroid and proteins, and each was extracted into a separate test tube with 1 ml of buffer containing a different concentration of KCl, from 0 to 0.6 M. The ^{3}H-steroid remaining on each filter and in an aliquot of each extract was then determined by scintillation spectrometry. Other aliquots of the extracts were treated with dextran-coated charcoal or analyzed by gel electrophoresis, gel filtration or density gradient centrifugation. When the salt concentration of the extracting buffer was low, the yield of ^{3}H-steroid-receptor complex was increased by a second extraction.

Results from this type of experiment with ^{3}H-progesterone-labelled chick oviduct cytosol are shown in Fig 8a. It is apparent that the steroid removed from the filter by each salt concentration was recovered nearly quantitatively in the extract. The maximal yield in the combined first and second extracts was obtained with 0.4 to 0.6 M KCl, and the half-maximal yield with 0.2 M KCl. The elution profile of progesterone receptors from DEAE filters was not simply a function of ionic strength, but showed some specificity with respect to the salt. Thus, the half-maximal elution occurred at 0.025 M $CaCl_2$, corresponding to a much lower ionic strength than 0.2 M KCl. In analogous experiments with ^{3}H-cortisol-labelled chick serum, half-maximal elution was obtained with 0.07 M KCl (13). This difference between the salt concentrations needed to elute the intracellular and serum complexes indicated the applicability of DEAE filters to the rapid fractionation of mixtures of steroid-binding components in small samples (e.g., 0.1 ml).

Schrader and O'Malley (14) showed that the major subcomponents of the chick oviduct progesterone receptor (labelled III and II in Fig 7a) could be eluted from DEAE-cellulose columns by 0.15 and

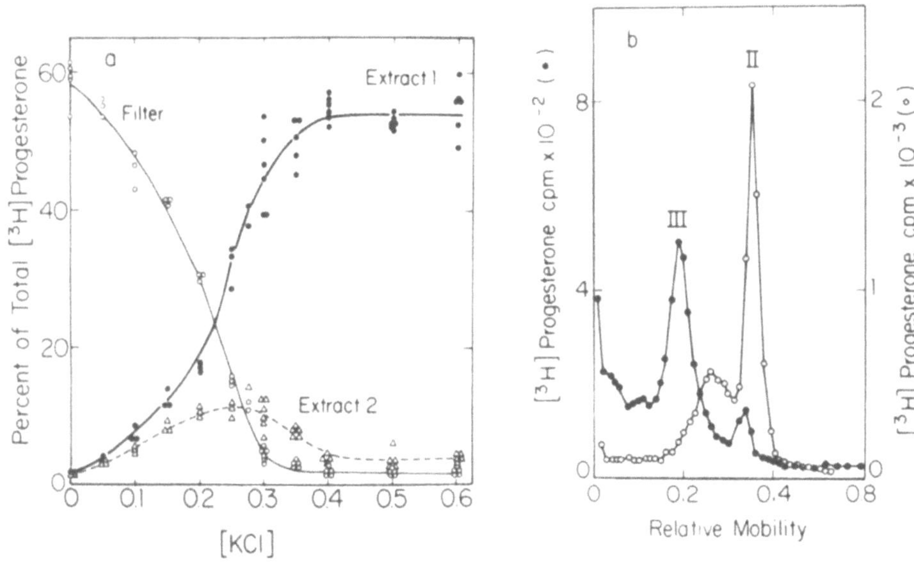

Fig 8. Preparative Ion Exchange Filtration of Progesterone Receptor Forms. (a) ^{3}H-Progesterone-labelled chick oviduct cytosol (0.1 ml) was adsorbed to DEAE filters on a manifold; unbound steroid and proteins were removed by five 1-ml washes with Tes-thioglycerol. Labelled complexes were extracted twice with 1 ml of Tes-thioglycerol containing 5 mg ovalbumin/ml (TTO) and the indicated KCl concentrations. (b) Labelled cytosol (0.1 ml) was adsorbed to filters and washed as in (a). Each filter was extracted four times with 0.5 ml of 0.15 M KCl in TTO, then with 0.5 ml of 0.35 M KCl in TTO. Aliquots (0.15 ml) of the first 0.15 M KCl extract (•) and the subsequent 0.35 M KCl extract (o) were electrophoresed on 15% C, 7% T polyacrylamide gels. Data from (13) and unpublished.

0.3 M KCl, respectively. We have used gel electrophoresis and gel filtration to characterize the complexes extracted from DEAE filters. The electrophoretic patterns in Fig 8b were obtained in 15% C, 7% T gels as described by Miller et al (5). The labelled complex in the 0.15 M KCl filter extract (III) appeared to migrate as a sharper peak and with a slightly lower mobility than the slow components of unfractionated cytosol under the same conditions (cf. Fig 6). The major component (II) in the 0.35 M KCl filter extract, following extraction with 0.15 M KCl, was indistinguishable from the fast component of cytosol (Fig 6) or from the complex in pool II from gel filtration analyzed under the same conditions. (Fig 7b shows the pattern in a 5% T gel).

Parallel studies were performed on the filter extracts by gel filtration. For these experiments (Fig 9a), the concentration of KCl in the high salt filter extract was increased from 0.35 to 0.5 M.

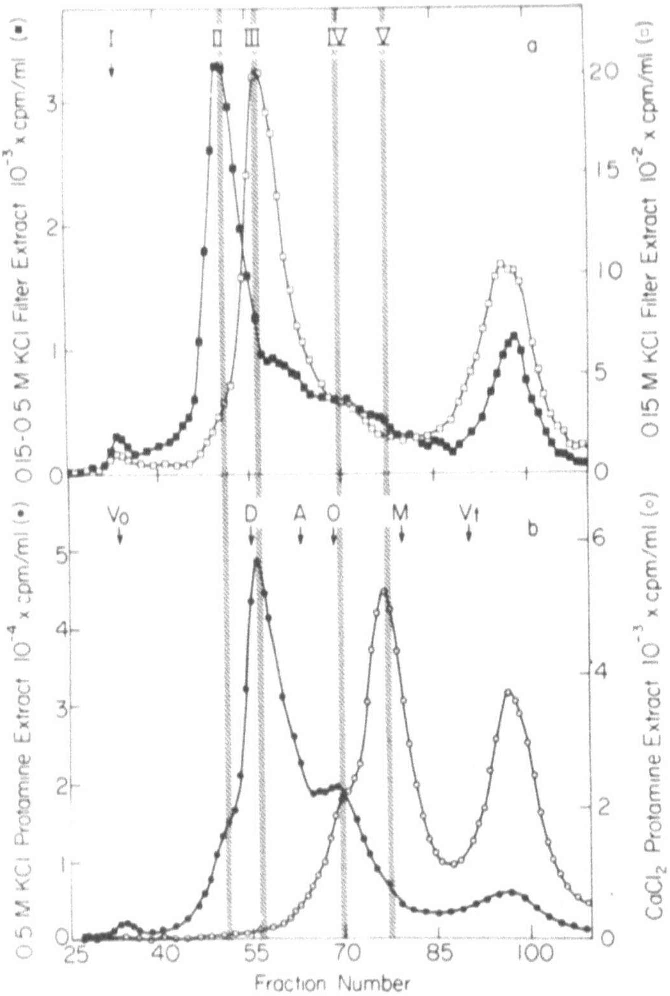

Fig 9. Gel Filtration of Progesterone Receptors Extracted from DEAE Filters or Protamine Precipitates (13). (a) ^{3}H-Progesterone-labelled cytosol was adsorbed to DEAE filters, washed, and extracted sequentially with 0.15 M (□) and 0.5 M KCl (■), as in Fig 8. Pooled extracts from two filters (0.8 ml) were chromatographed as in Fig 7a. (b) Receptors were precipitated from 1 ml of cytosol with 940µg of protamine sulfate, washed, and extracted with 1 ml of 0.5 M KCl or 20mM $CaCl_2$ (16). Elution patterns of 0.9 ml of the KCl extract (•) and 0.37 ml of the $CaCl_2$ extract (o) are shown. The void volume (V_o), total liquid volume (V_t), and elution volumes of receptor aggregates (I), the major receptor forms (II,III,V), a minor complex in protamine extracts (IV), myoglobin (M), ovalbumin (O), albumin monomer (A) and dimer (D) are shown.

This did not alter the shape of the gel filtration or polyacrylamide gel patterns, but improved the yield of the labelled complex. The conclusion from both the chromatographic and electrophoretic analyses was that the DEAE filters permitted the rapid and effective separation of the two major subcomponents of this receptor (II and III in Figs 8b and 9a).

Another technique that has been useful in analyzing the substructure of progesterone receptors is precipitation with polyamines such as protamine sulfate (15) or polylysine, and extraction of the pellets with solutions of various salts. Sherman et al (16) showed that the complex extracted from protamine-precipitated cytosol by $CaCl_2$ had a sedimentation coefficient of only 2.5 S, compared with 3.5 S for the KCl extract. Gel electrophoresis (13) and agarose gel filtration showed that the KCl protamine extract contained only one of the major forms observed in whole cytosol under these conditions (III in Figs 7a and 9b). In contrast, gel filtration of the $CaCl_2$ protamine extract revealed a major component (V) that co-chromatographed with the standard protein myoglobin (M in Fig 9b). Since this 20,000 molecular weight complex is the smallest subunit or fragment of the receptor containing the specific high-affinity steroid-binding site, it has been called the steroid-binding "subunit" (16) or the mero-receptor (13). From a combination of the sedimentation coefficient and the Stokes radius, determined by gel filtration (2), the mero-receptor was calculated to be a globular protein (axial ratio$\sim$1). Analogous calculations for components II and III gave axial ratios of 8 to 12 (13).

Recently, the direct conversion of component II to the mero-receptor was accomplished by incubating the 0.15 to 0.5 M KCl extract from DEAE filters with 20mM $CaCl_2$ for 2 hrs at 4 C (M.R. Sherman and S.C. Diaz, in preparation). The dramatic decrease in the axial ratio of the labelled complex during $CaCl_2$-treatment suggests that an asymmetric polypeptide was released. New techniques must now be developed to detect and isolate the part of the receptor that does not appear to be involved in steroid-binding but may be essential for the interaction with chromatin.

SUMMARY

Many studies of steroid receptors in amphibian, avian and mammalian target organs have consisted of: 1) the evaluation of binding parameters (specificity, affinity, capacity) by incubation with a ^{3}H-steroid and removal of free ^{3}H-steroid by adsorption to charcoal or gel filtration, and 2) determination of the sedimentation coefficients of the complexes in cytoplasmic and/or nuclear extracts by density gradient centrifugation. In this chapter, we have surveyed a number of additional techniques that can be used both to fractionate mixtures of steroid-binding proteins and to evaluate their molecular weights, Stokes radii, axial ratios and relative net charges. Analyses of competitive steroid binding by techniques that discriminate not only between bound and free steroid but among several steroid-binding proteins were exemplified by gel filtration and electrophoretic patterns for human breast tumor cytosol and serum (Figs 1-4). The advantages of fractionating steroid receptors and other proteins by electrophoresis in gels of large but varied pore size were shown in Figs 5 and 6.

Studies of the multiple forms of the chick oviduct progesterone receptor served to illustrate some useful combinations of techniques: electrophoresis following gel filtration (Fig 7) or elution from DEAE filters (Fig 8), and gel filtration following protamine precipitation or ion exchange filtration (Fig 9). Although the first step in each sequence was performed on unfractionated cytosol, the results permitted a detailed comparison of the molecular parameters of the major subcomponents of the receptor (II and III in Figs 7-9), and the smaller steroid-binding unit (V in Fig 9). Thus, form II has the largest Stokes radius, highest axial ratio and highest net negative charge in the pH range of 7.4 to 10.2. A lower net negative charge on form III accounts for its lower electrophoretic mobility in gels (despite its smaller radius) and its greater ease of extraction from DEAE-cellulose or protamine precipitates (13). Recently, another combination of techniques permitted the demonstration that form II, but not form III, prepared by ion exchange filtration, is converted to form V on exposure to $CaCl_2$ (M.R. Sherman and S.C. Diaz, in preparation).

ACKNOWLEDGMENTS

We are grateful to Soledad Diaz and Fe Tuazon for their skillful participation in many of these experiments, to the Tumor Procurement Service of Memorial Hospital for providing breast tumors and blood, to Drs. Celia Menendes-Botet and Jerome Nisselbaum for preparing tumor cytosol, to Drs. Andreas Chrambach and David Rodbard for invaluable advice concerning electrophoresis and to Dr. John L. Lewis, Jr., for research facilities and funds. This investigation was supported in part by National Institutes of Health Grants CA-16814, CA-08748 and HL-06285, American Cancer Society Grant PRA-83, and the Paul Garrett Fund.

REFERENCES

1. Sherman, M.R., P.L. Corvol and B.W. O'Malley, J. Biol. Chem. 245:6085, 1970.

2. Sherman, M.R., Methods Enzymol. 36:211, 1975.

3. Mickelson, K.E. and P.H. Petra, Biochemistry 14:957, 1975.

4. Corvol, P.L., A. Chrambach, D. Rodbard and C.W. Bardin, J. Biol. Chem. 246:3435, 1971.

5. Miller, L.K., S.C. Diaz and M.R. Sherman, Biochemistry 14: 4433, 1975.

6. Davis, B.J., Ann. N.Y. Acad. Sci. 121:404, 1964.

7. Rodbard, D., C. Levitov and A. Chrambach, Sep. Sci. 7:705, 1972.

8. Ferguson, K.A., Metabolism 13:985, 1964.

9. Chrambach, A. and D. Rodbard, Science 172:440, 1971.

10. Rodbard, D. and A. Chrambach, Anal. Biochem. 40:95, 1971.

11. Rodbard, D. and A. Chrambach, In: Allen, R.C. and H.R. Maurer (eds.), Electrophoresis and Isoelectric Focusing on Polyacrylamide Gel, Walter de Gruyter, Berlin, 1974, p. 28.

12. Santi, D.V., C.H. Sibley, E.R. Perriard, G.M. Tomkins and J.D. Baxter, Biochemistry 12:2412, 1973.

13. Sherman, M.R., F.B. Tuazon, S.C. Diaz and L.K. Miller, Biochemistry 15:980, 1976.

14. Schrader, W.T. and B.W. O'Malley, J. Biol. Chem. 247:51, 1972.

15. King, R.J.B., J. Gordon and A.W. Steggles, Biochem. J. 114: 649, 1969.

16. Sherman, M.R., S.B.P. Atienza, J.R. Shansky and L.M. Hoffman, J. Biol. Chem. 249:5351, 1974.

MAMMALIAN PROGESTERONE RECEPTORS: BIOSYNTHESIS, STRUCTURE AND NUCLEAR BINDING

L.E. Faber*, J. Saffran*, T.J. Chen** and W.W. Leavitt**

*Endocrine Research Unit
Medical College of Ohio, Toledo, Ohio
**Department of Physiology
University of Cincinnati College of Medicine
Cincinnati, Ohio

Because estrogen and progesterone receptors may be involved in the endocrine sensitivity of certain breast and endometrial carcinomas (1,2), considerable interest has been generated in the study of steroid receptors in hormonally sensitive tumors. In this chapter, we will review some recent progress on three aspects of receptor biology as applied to mammalian progesterone receptors: regulation of receptor biosynthesis, structure of the receptor and nuclear binding of the steroid-receptor complex.

REGULATION OF PROGESTERONE RECEPTOR SYNTHESIS BY ESTROGEN

In vivo studies have demonstrated that the progesterone-binding capacity of uterus (3,4) and vagina (4) is stimulated by estrogen. Although it has been recognized for some time that prior estrogen action is necessary for progestational responses, the mechanism is not well understood. Estrogen-mediated stimulation of progesterone receptor formation offers one possible explanation.

Studies with the guinea pig (5), rat and mouse (6) and hamster (7) indicated that the concentrations of uterine progesterone-binding components varied during the reproductive cycle. During the 4-day hamster estrous cycle, cellular concentrations of receptor increased during diestrus and reached a peak at proestrus, corresponding to the increase in serum estradiol levels (7). Formation of the 6-7S progesterone binding component occurred during the follicular phase of the cycle. The uterine progesterone receptor concentration

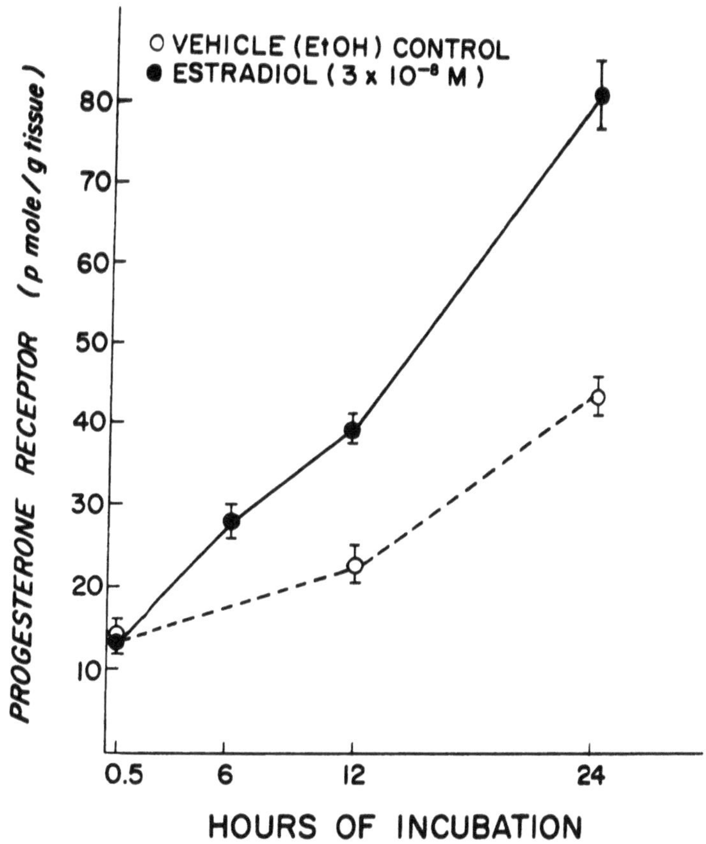

Fig 1. Progesterone Receptor Production by Hamster Uterine Strips During Incubation at 37C. Open circles represent control strips which were exposed to ethanol vehicle (3μl/4ml medium 199) during preincubation. Estradiol-17β treated strips (closed circles) were preincubated with estradiol-17β for 1 hr at 25C. Each point represents the mean ± S.E.M. progesterone receptor concentration.

decreased slowly following ovariectomy at proestrus, and was rapidly restored by estrogen treatment. These results supported the idea that estrogen action during the cycle promoted formation of the progesterone receptor.

In the hamster, progesterone treatment given early on the day of proestrus caused a rapid premature depletion of receptor from the cytosol fraction (7,8). Cellular concentrations of receptor dropped markedly between proestrus and estrus, corresponding to the time of preovulatory progesterone secretion (7). Thus, variations in progesterone receptor levels during the female cycle may be attributed to the cyclic pattern of estrogen and progestin secretion.

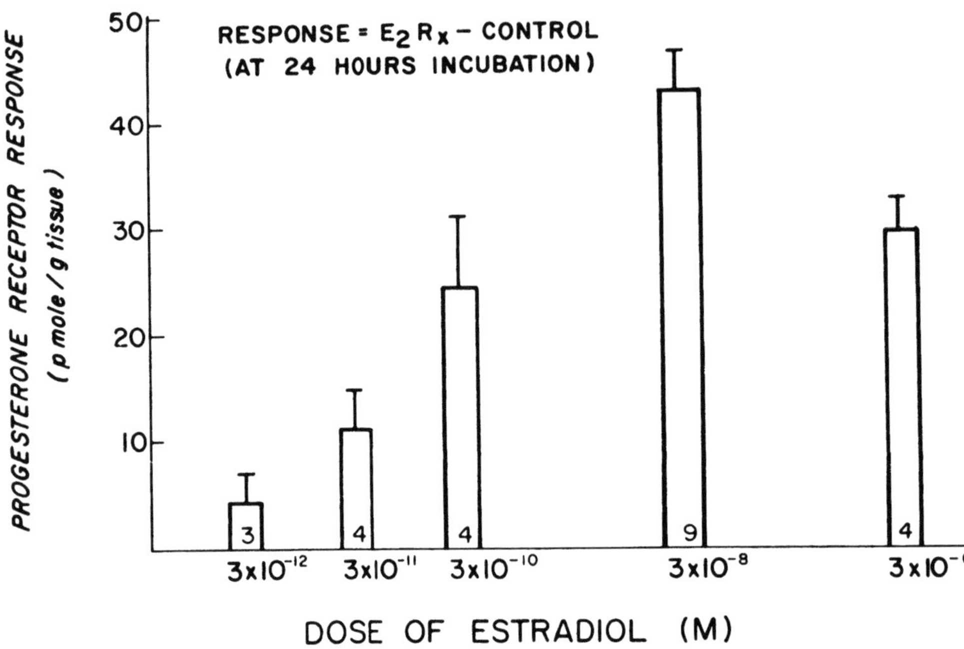

Fig 2. Responsiveness of Hamster Uterine Strips to Estrogen In Vitro. Uterine strips were exposed to different concentrations of estradiol-17β during preincubation. The results present the increment of progesterone receptor production comparing estradiol-treated (E_2R_X) and control strips. Each bar is the mean $\pm$ S.E.M. of 3 or more observations.

The estrogen-induction of the progesterone receptors appears to involve RNA and protein synthesis. Administration of actinomycin D or cycloheximide just before estrogen treatment (ovariectomized guinea pig) prevented receptor formation in the uterus (9). Similar results were obtained with the hamster (10,11). These findings support the hypothesis that estrogen increases the production of progesterone receptor molecules via stimulation of RNA and protein synthesis. However, additional studies were necessary to establish that estrogen stimulated *de novo* progesterone receptor synthesis, as opposed to an activation of precursor molecules. An *in vitro* incubation system using uterine tissue derived from ovariectomized hamsters (10 days after ovariectomy) was developed to test this hypothesis (12). Uterine strips were prepared and placed in 25 ml flasks containing 4 ml of medium 199 (Gibco). Paired flasks received equivalent amounts (110-120 mg) of tissue from each donor animal. Uterine strips were preincubated with estradiol-17β or ethanol vehicle (3µl/4ml medium 199) at 25C for 1 hr. Then, the strips were rinsed in fresh medium and incubated in hormone-free medium 199 under an atmosphere of 95% O_2 and 5% CO_2. At the end of

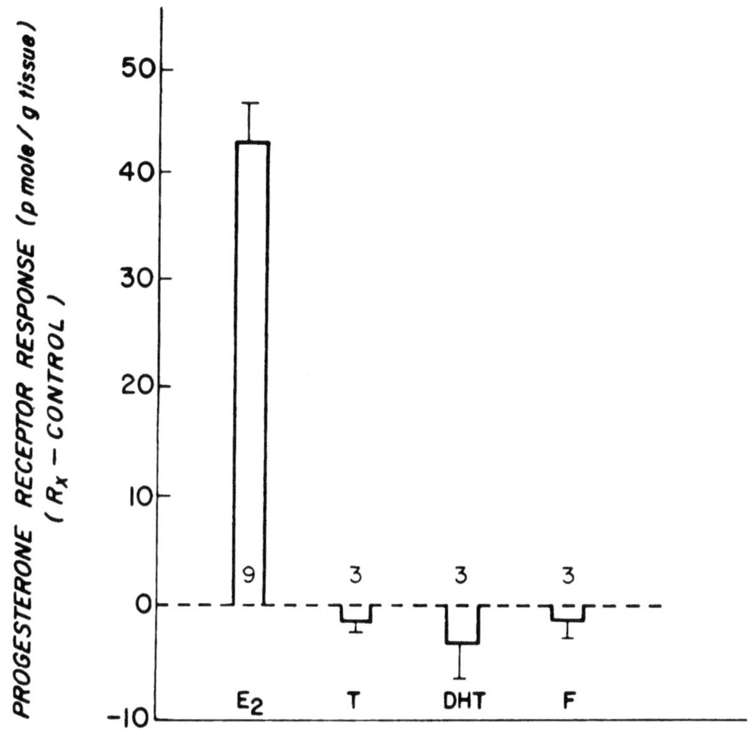

Fig 3. Specificity of Progesterone Receptor Response to Estrogen. Hamster uterine strips were preincubated with 3 x 10^{-8}M estradiol-17β (E_2), testosterone (T), 5α-dihydrotestosterone (DHT) or cortisol (F). The results represent the difference in progesterone receptor production comparing steroid-treated (R_x) and control strips. Each bar is the mean ± S.E.M., and the number of observations is indicated.

the incubation, uterine strips were removed, chilled and the cytosol fraction prepared as described elsewhere (7). The receptor concentration (pmole/g tissue) was measured in the cytosol fraction by Scatchard analysis of specific ^{3}H-progesterone binding (7).

First, the time course of *in vitro* receptor production by uterine strips was studied (Fig 1). The initial progesterone receptor concentration in fresh uterine tissue was 30 ± 2.1 pmole/gm tissue. Substantial amounts of receptor appeared to be lost during preparation and preincubation of the strips. However, controls showed increased receptor levels during incubation from 0.5 hrs to 24 hrs (Fig 1). *In vitro* estradiol-17β treatment significantly enhanced receptor production at 6, 12 and 24 hrs.

The responsiveness of the *in vitro* system to estrogen was evaluated by a dose-response study. Uterine strips were exposed to

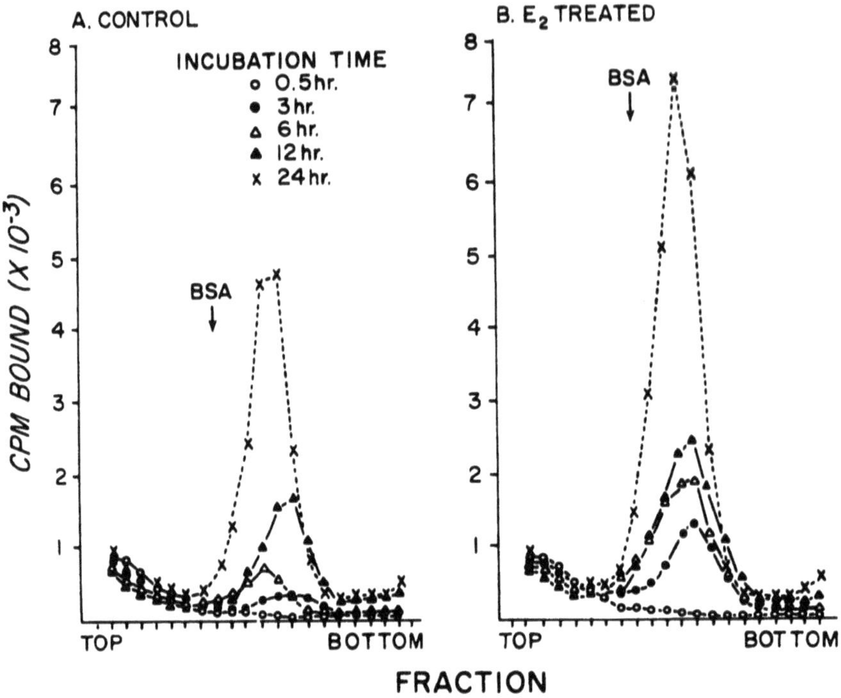

Fig 4. Sedimentation Properties of Progesterone Receptor Produced In Vitro. Hamster uterine cytosols were labelled with ^{3}H-progesterone and assayed by sucrose density gradient centrifugation as described elsewhere (6). Free or loosely bound progesterone was removed from each gradient fraction using dextran-coated charcoal. The sedimentation peak of the bovine serum albumin (BSA) standard (4.6S) is indicated by the arrow. A. Control strips were exposed to ethanol vehicle during preincubation. B. Estradiol-17β (E_2) treated uterine strips were preincubated with 3 x 10^{-8}M E_2 for 1 hr at 25C.

increasing concentrations of estradiol (3 x 10^{-12}M to 3 x 10^{-6}M) during preincubation. A significant receptor response was obtained with 3 x 10^{-11}M estradiol (Fig 2), and a maximal response occurred after incubation in 3 x 10^{-8}M estradiol.

It was important to determine whether the induction of the progesterone receptor could be mediated by estrogen receptors. If so, the amount of estrogen needed to induce the progesterone receptor should approximate the amount of available estrogen receptor, and the induction of progesterone receptor should be specific for estrogen. Scatchard analysis of ^{3}H-estradiol-17β binding in untreated uterine strips revealed 7.1 $\pm$ 0.3 pmole estradiol-17β binding sites/gm tissue (about 0.8 pmole of estrogen receptor/flask). A half-maximal progesterone receptor response was achieved with 3 x 10^{-10}M estradiol-17β (1.2 pmole estradiol-17β/flask) (Fig 2).

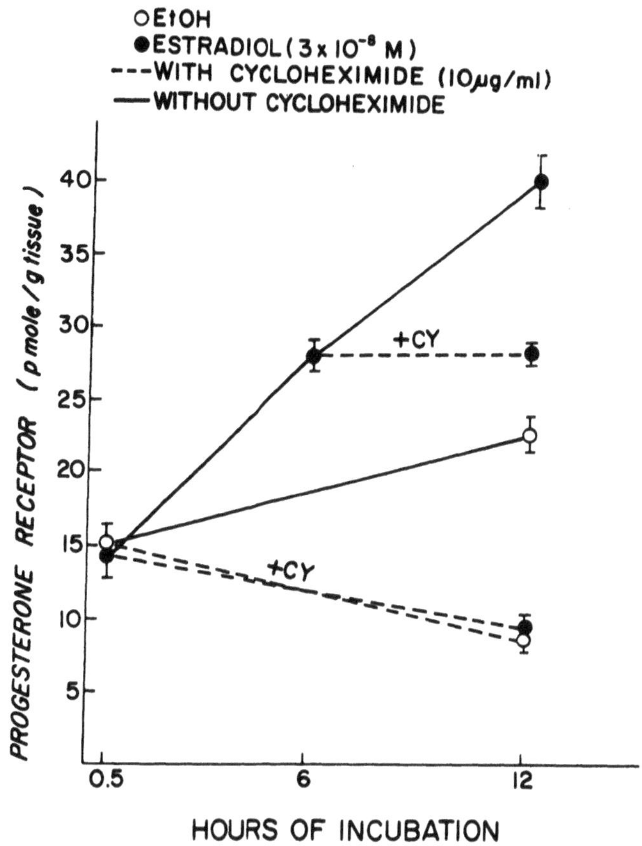

Fig 5. Dependence of Progesterone Receptor Production on Protein Synthesis. Control strips (open circles) were exposed to ethanol vehicle during preincubation. Closed circles represent strips pretreated with 3 x 10^{-8}M estradiol-17β for 1 hr at 25C. Cycloheximide (CY) treatment (10μg/ml) (dashed line) before incubation abolished receptor production in both control and estrogen-treated hamster uterine strips, while CY treatment at 6 hr prevented receptor synthesis from 6 to 12 hrs. Each point represents the mean ± S.E.M. of 3 or more observations.

Thus, there was agreement between the concentration of estrogen needed to induce the progesterone receptor and the amount of estrogen receptor in the tissue.

Additional evidence indicating a role of the estrogen receptor in induction of progesterone receptor formation was provided by a specificity study. Uterine strips were exposed to different hormonal steroids (3 x 10^{-8}M) during preincubation. Subsequent incubation

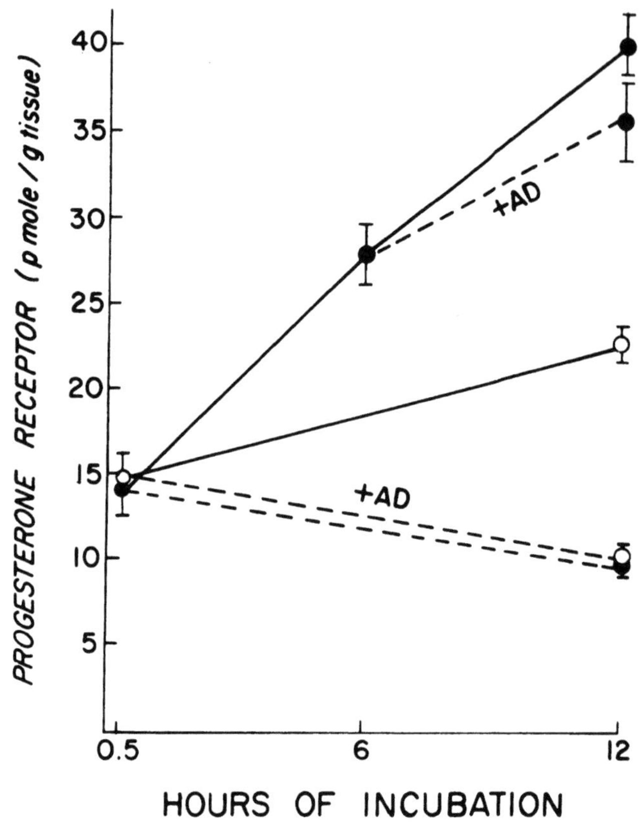

Fig 6. Dependence of Progesterone Receptor Production on RNA Synthesis. Actinomycin D (AD) treatment (10μg/ml) (dashed line) before incubation blocked progesterone receptor production in both control (open circles) and estrogen-treated uterine strips (closed circles). However, AD given at 6 hr to estrogen-treated strips did not inhibit subsequent receptor synthesis.

at 37C revealed that synthesis was increased only by estradiol. No effect on progesterone receptor induction was observed after treatment with testosterone (T), 5α-dihydrotestosterone (DHT) or cortisol (F) (Fig 3).

The sedimentation coefficient of the progesterone receptor produced during incubation of control and estrogen-treated uterine strips was determined by density-gradient centrifugation. The receptor synthesized by both control and estrogen-treated strips had a sedimentation coefficient of 6-7S in low ionic strength medium (Fig 4). The size of the 7S peak increased with the time of incu-

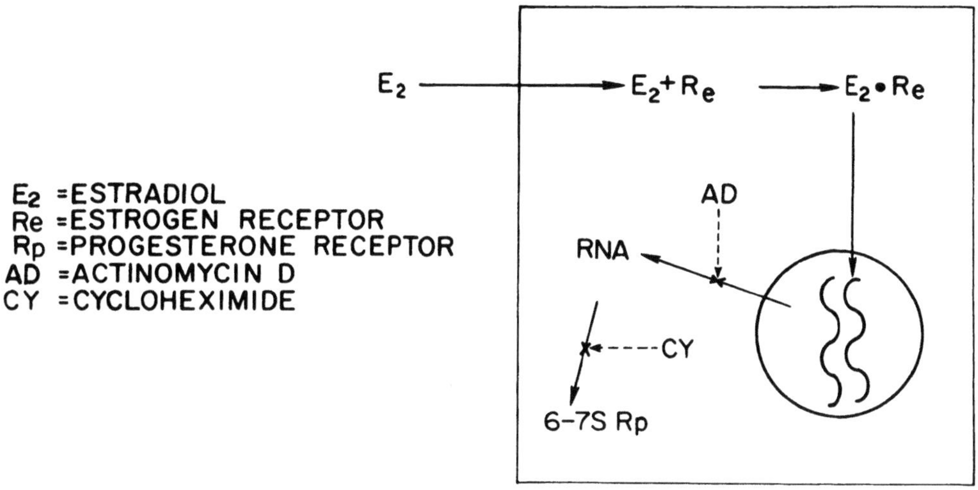

Fig 7. Proposed Mechanism of Progesterone Receptor Synthesis in Uterine Tissue. Progesterone receptor is synthesized without estrogen support. This is dependent on RNA and protein synthesis and may be blocked by actinomycin D (AD) and cycloheximide (CY). Estradiol-17β (E_2) increases progesterone receptor synthesis via stimulation of RNA and protein synthesis. Estradiol appears to enhance receptor synthesis via the estrogen receptor system.

bation in both groups. More 7S receptor was found in the estrogen-treated strips. This finding was consistent with the measurements of progesterone binding capacity. Other workers had suggested that a smaller (4S) form of receptor might be produced during the early stages of estrogen action (9,13). Present *in vitro* studies with hamster uterus failed to demonstrate a 4S progesterone-binding component during early estrogen action. These results suggest that the 4S component may be a serum protein which accumulates in the uterus because of the hyperemic response to estrogen (10,12).

Cycloheximide, a protein synthesis inhibitor, has been employed to study the involvement of protein synthesis in the production of the progesterone receptor. Treatment of uterine strips with cycloheximide (10μg/ml) during incubation blocked receptor synthesis (Fig 5). Exposure of estrogen-treated strips to cycloheximide (10μg/ml) after a 6 hr incubation, also inhibited receptor synthesis. Thus, it would appear that estrogen-stimulated receptor production is dependent on continued protein synthesis throughout the time course of the response.

Similar studies were performed using actinomycin D to determine whether progesterone receptor synthesis was dependent on RNA synthesis. Addition of actinomycin D (10μg/ml) to the incubation media blocked subsequent receptor production in both control and estrogen-treated strips (Fig 6). However, when estrogen-treated strips were exposed to actinomycin D after 6 hr of incubation, receptor synthesis was not inhibited. This suggested that enough estrogen-dependent RNA was produced during the first six hours of estrogen action to sustain receptor synthesis in the absence of new RNA synthesis.

Results obtained with uterine strips support the following model of progesterone receptor synthesis (Fig 7). The basal level of progesterone receptor synthesis is dependent on RNA and protein synthesis. Interaction of estradiol with its receptor causes translocation of the estrogen receptor complex to nuclear acceptor sites and stimulate RNA synthesis. The increase in estrogen dependent RNA results in an accelerated synthesis of the progesterone receptor.

THE STRUCTURE OF THE MAMMALIAN PROGESTERONE RECEPTOR

Work on the structure of steroid receptors has been hampered by low concentrations of receptor and by the fact that receptors are detectable only when complexed with a radioactive hormone. The steroid-receptor complex may be viewed as a functional unit, composed of several subunits. The concentrations of these subunits may vary with the physiological state of the cell. Sometime in the future it should be possible to identify the receptor configuration in the cell and thereby gain much information about the physiological or pathological state of the cell. The problem facing the biochemist is to correctly identify the structure of the molecule and then attribute a biological function to each form of the receptor.

The receptor forms can be placed in three classes on the basis of sedimentation coefficient. The largest complex, 7S, presumably contains all of the functional units. In solutions of 300mM KCl or other media of high ionic strength it is replaced by one or more 4S species. Under certain conditions, the 4S form may be converted to the 7S complex by removal of salt. A third form, of intermediate sedimentation coefficient (5.5 to 6.0S), has been implicated in nuclear binding. The relationships among these receptor forms are under intense study.

TABLE 1

Comparison of the Half-Life of the 7S Uterine Progesterone Receptor in Two Buffering Solutions

Buffering Solution	Composition	Half-Life (Hrs) Rabbit	Guinea Pig
TGE	10mM TRIS-HCl, 10% glycerol, 1.5mM Na_2 EDTA	24	54
5mM PGT	5mM Sodium Phosphate, 10% glycerol, 10mM Monothioglycerol-degassed	176	192

With respect to mammalian progesterone receptors it is possible to stabilize either the 4S or 7S complex. A partial stabilization of the 7S progesterone receptor complex from guinea pig and rabbit uterus has recently been achieved (14) (Table 1).

In these experiments uterine cytosols of either rabbit or guinea pig were prepared in the designated buffer solution. Aliquots of the ^{3}H-progesterone labelled cytosol were sedimented through 5-20% sucrose gradients immediately after preparation, or after storage for several days at 4C. The half-life of the receptor complex in a particular solution was estimated by plotting the decay of the 7S material as a function of time. In the commonly used TGE (10mM TRIS-HCl, 10% glycerol (V/V), 1.5mM Na_2 EDTA, pH 7.4) buffer, the half-life of the rabbit uterine 7S receptor was about 24 hrs, and that of the guinea pig roughly 54 hrs. Another buffering solution, 5mM PGT (5mM sodium phosphate, 10% glycerol (V/V), 10mM monothioglycerol, which is degassed, pH 7.4), was also tested. In this solution the half-life of the rabbit uterine 7S complex was approximately 176 hrs and that of the guinea pig about 192 hrs. These data illustrate the influence of the buffer constituents on the stability of a specific receptor form.

In addition to effects on sedimentation behavior, the ionic composition of the buffering medium appears to alter the steroid-binding properties of the receptor. Scatchard analyses or equilibrium dialysis experiments carried out in 300mM KCl and 100mM sodium phosphate are presented in Table 2. The apparent association constant "K_a" for progesterone binding by either rabbit or guinea pig uterine cytosol was about 1 to 2 x $10^9 M^{-1}$. Addition of potas-

TABLE 2

EFFECT OF 300mM KCl and 100mM SODIUM PHOSPHATE ON THE APPARENT ASSOCIATION CONSTANT OF THE BINDING OF 1,2,6,7-^{3}H-PROGESTERONE BY GUINEA PIG AND RABBIT UTERINE CYTOSOL

Buffering Solution	Apparent Association Constant(M^{-1})[1] Rabbit	Guinea Pig
5mM PGT	1.1×10^9	1.0×10^9
5mM PGT + 300mM KCl[2]	0.5×10^9	0.5×10^9
100mM PGT[3]	2.3×10^9	1.2×10^9

[1] Estimates of "K_a" were made utilizing the Ellis-Kersco equilibrium dialysis method previously described (15). The cytosol protein concentration was 5mg/ml and dialysis was for 24 hrs at 4C.

[2] 5mM sodium phosphate, 10% glycerol, 10mM monothioglycerol + 300mM KCl-degassed (pH 7.4).

[3] 100mM sodium phosphate, 10% glycerol, 10mM monothioglycerol-degassed (pH 7.4).

sium chloride (300mM) reduced the binding constant by roughly one-half. This is not a general salt effect because increasing the concentration of sodium phosphate to 100mM did not depress the "K_a". Therefore, it appears that it is possible to modify the binding characteristics of the receptor by use of certain salts.

Stabilization of the 7S uterine progesterone receptor has permitted chromatography of uterine cytosols. The behavior of the receptor has been studied by filtration through various gels. An example is presented in Fig 8. In this experiment guinea pig uterine cytosol was incubated with ^{3}H-progesterone and chromatographed through a Sephadex G-200 column. This column was eluted with high ionic strength phosphate buffer (100mM PGT). A single peak of tritium migrated just behind the void volume (Fig 8A). Density gradient centrifugation of the material in the peak revealed a 4.5S binder in high ionic strength solutions (100mM PGT) and a 5.5S complex in low ionic strength media (5mM PGT). Because little 7S binding was found, various fractions of the column eluate were combined. Assay of the material in the ascending limb of the peak (Pool 1), added to faster migrating fractions, once again yielded 4.5S binding in high salt and 5.5S binding in low salt (Fig 8B). However, when

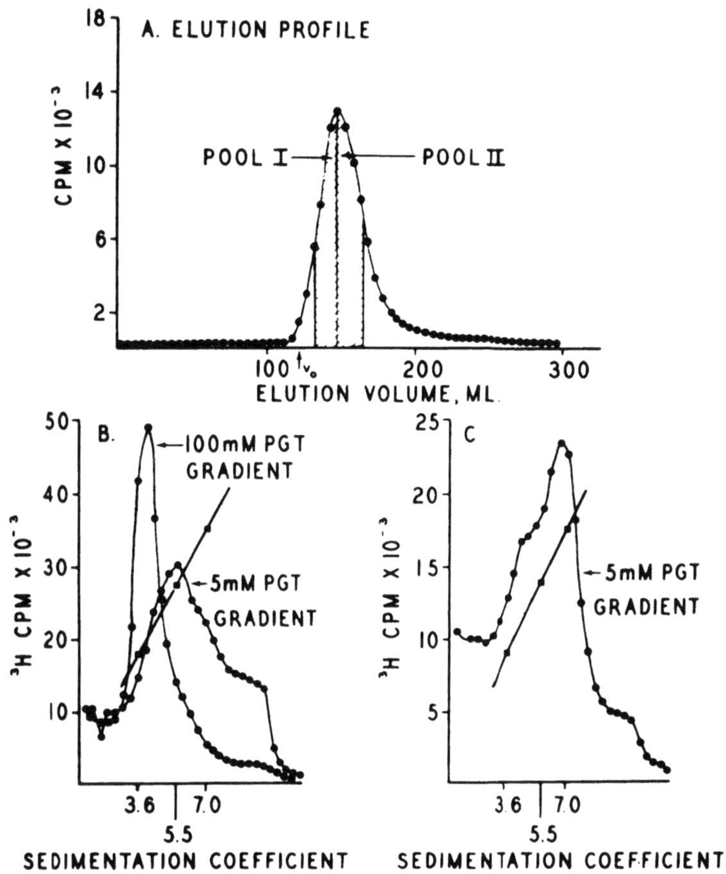

Fig 8. Chromatography of Guinea Pig Uterine Cytosol Labelled with ^{3}H-Progesterone. A. Elution profile of G-200 column eluted with high ionic strength buffer (100mM PGT). B. Sucrose density gradient centrifugation of Pool I, to which had been added the faster migrating fractions, through sucrose gradients made up in 5mM PGT or 100mM PGT. C. Sucrose density gradient centrifugation of Pool II to which had been added fractions which were retarded on the column. The diagonal straight line in B and C is a plot of the sedimentation coefficients for protein markers used as standards.

the material in the descending limb (Pool II) was added to the material which had been retarded by the column, formation of the 7S complex (Fig 8C) could be demonstrated. Data of this nature suggest that there are three basic forms of the receptor (4.5S, 5.5S and 7S) and indicate that there may be a subunit structure to the receptor. In the case of the progesterone receptor, it appears that the 5.5S form may be derived directly from the 7S complex, in low ionic strength media. The smallest progesterone receptor complex of mammalian uteri (4.5S) is usually seen under conditions of high ionic strength. Clarification of the interconversions of the various forms of the receptor should lead to better understanding of the role of the receptors in steroid hormone action.

NUCLEAR BINDING OF THE PROGESTERONE RECEPTOR

Experimental evidence indicates that the specificity of nuclear binding of progesterone in the rabbit and guinea pig uterus resides in the cytoplasmic receptor. Cytosols of estrogen stimulated uteri allowed progesterone to be bound by isolated nuclei, but cytosols of non-target tissues or of unstimulated uteri were not effective in promoting nuclear uptake (Fig 9A). However, nuclei of estrogen-stimulated and unstimulated uteri bound progesterone equally well, and non-target tissue nuclei also bound progesterone (Fig 9B).

The rate of nuclear binding depends upon the temperature of the incubation. At 0C the binding was very slow but increasing the temperature to 20C increased the rate of binding (Fig 10). At 20C the amount of receptor in the cytosol decreased as the amount bound

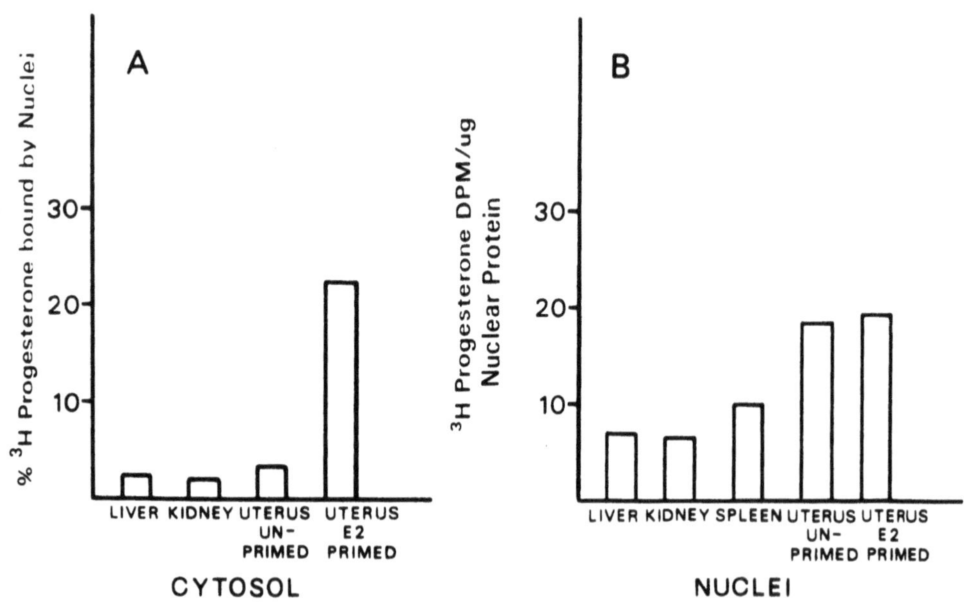

Fig 9. Specificity of ^{3}H-Progesterone Uptake by Rabbit Uterine Nuclei. A. Effect of cytosols. B. Effect of nuclear preparations of various tissues. Incubations were carried out at 20C for 60 minutes.

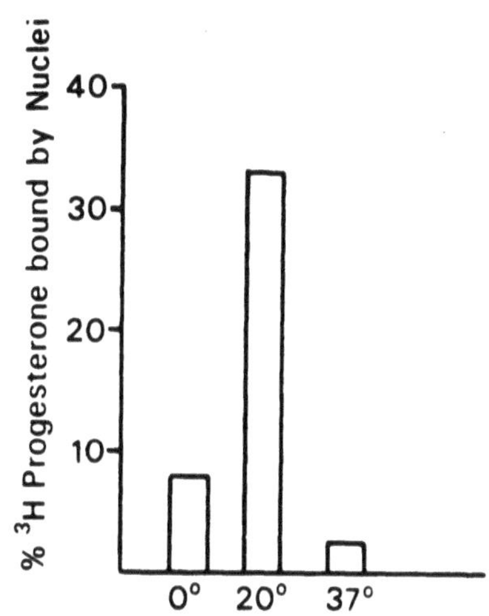

Fig 10. Effect of Incubation Temperature on the Uptake of ^{3}H-Progesterone by Guinea Pig Uterine Nuclei. Incubations were carried out for 60 minutes at the temperature indicated.

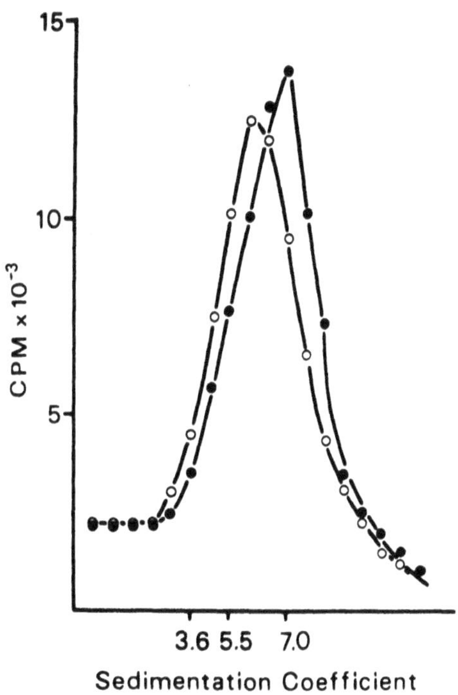

Fig 11. Sucrose Density Gradient Centrifugation of Guinea Pig Uterine Cytosol. Samples were diluted 1 to 2 and incubated with 1,2,6,7^{3}H-progesterone for 60 minutes at 0C (closed circles); or 30 minutes at 20C (open circles).

to nuclei increased. Nuclear binding at any temperature depends on a balance between binding rate and inactivation of the receptor. Between 0 and 25C, the receptor was stable enough so that the same degree of nuclear uptake was eventually reached. At 30C and especially at 37C the rate of inactivation exceeded the rate of binding.

Because of the effects of temperature on the nuclear uptake, the effect of temperature on the sedimentation properties of the cytoplasmic progesterone receptor was studied. When progesterone was incubated with guinea pig uterine cytosol at 0C, a binding peak with a sedimentation coefficient of 7S was seen. Dilution of the cytosol and incubation at 0C did not alter the sedimentation properties of the receptor. When the incubation was carried out at 20C the 7S peak became somewhat broader and a shoulder at 5S was sometimes seen. However, when the cytosol was diluted 1 in 2 with ^{3}H-progesterone at 20C, the sedimentation coefficient decreased to 5.5S (Fig 11). These data point to a shift in sedimentation coefficient of 7S to 5.5S under conditions paralleling nuclear uptake studies.

Guinea pig uterine cytosol, without added ^{3}H-progesterone, was chromatographed on Sephadex G-100. The fractions eluted from the

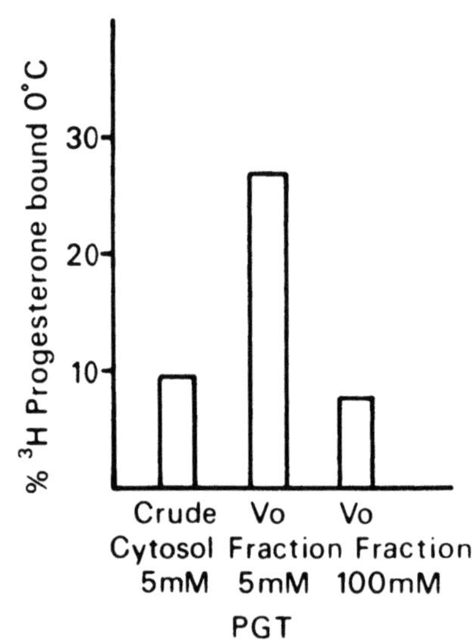

Fig 12. Nuclear Binding of Progesterone-Receptor Complex with Crude Guinea Pig Uterine Cytosol and with the V_o Fraction after Chromatography on Sephadex G-100. Nuclei were incubated with ^{3}H-progesterone and either cytosol or V_o fraction for 60 minutes at 0C. In some incubations the molarity of the PGT was adjusted to 100mM.

column were tested for their ability to bind ^{3}H-progesterone and to stimulate nuclear binding. The concentrated void volume fraction had a sedimentation coefficient of 5.5S on sucrose density gradient centrifugation in 5mM PGT or 4S in 100mM PGT. In the presence of crude cytosol uterine nuclei bound ^{3}H-progesterone very slowly at OC. But in the presence of the 5.5S fraction nuclear binding took place more rapidly at OC (Fig 12), once again implicating the 5.5S form of the receptor in nuclear binding. This 5.5S complex may be the receptor form which enters the nucleus, and the conversion of the 7S form of the receptor to the 5.5S complex may be one aspect of the "transformation" process.

ACKNOWLEDGMENTS

Supported in part by Grants M74.113; HD 06982, OCM 75-16135 (W.W.L.), HD 09367 (L.F.), and HD 09359 (J.S.) and Contracts HD-72-2710 and HD 4-2851 (L.F. and J.S.).

REFERENCES

1. Horwitz, K.B., W.L. McGuire, O.H. Pearson and A. Segaloff, Science 189:726, 1976.

2. Reel, J.R., In: Menon, K.M.J. and J.R. Reel (eds.), Steroid Hormone Action and Cancer, Plenum Press, New York, 1976, p. 85.

3. Falk, R.J. and C.W. Bardin, Endocrinology 86:1059, 1970.

4. Leavitt, W.W. and G.C. Blaha, Steroids 19:262, 1972.

5. Milgrom, E., M. Atger, M. Perrot and E.-E. Baulieu, Endocrinology 90:1071, 1972.

6. Feil, P.D., S.R. Glasser, D.O. Toft and B.W. O'Malley, Endocrinology 91:738, 1972.

7. Leavitt, W.W., D.O. Toft, C.A. Strott and B.W. O'Malley, Endocrinology 94:1041, 1974.

8. Leavitt, W.W. and C.J. Grossman, Proc. Natl. Acad. Sci., U.S.A. 71:4341, 1974.

9. Milgrom, E., L. Thi, M. Atger and E.-E. Baulieu, J. Biol. Chem. 248:6366, 1973.

10. Chen, T.J. and W.W. Leavitt, Fed. Proc. 34:279, 1975.

11. Reel, J.R. and Y. Shih, Acta Endocr. 80:344, 1975.

12. Chen, T.J. and W.W. Leavitt, Physiologist 18:166, 1975.

13. Toft, D.O. and B.W. O'Malley, Endocrinology 90:1041, 1972.

14. Faber, L.E., M.L. Sandmann and H.E. Stavely, Fed. Proc. 22: 229, 1973.

15. Faber, L.E., M.L. Sandmann and H.E. Stavely, J. Biol. Chem. 247:8000, 1972.

THE MODE OF ACTION OF PROGESTAGENS ON ENDOMETRIAL CARCINOMA

Jerry R. Reel

Department of Pharmacology
Parke, Davis & Company
Ann Arbor, Michigan

Buoyed by the beneficial effects of endocrine therapy in prostate and breast cancer, Kelley and Baker (1) in 1951 began treating patients with metastatic or recurrent endometrial carcinoma with progestational compounds. By the late 1950's and early 1960's several other clinicians also were using progestagens to treat selected cases of endometrial carcinoma (2-9). From the data that have accumulated, it appears that *remission** of the disease occurs in about 30-35% of the treated patients (1,10,11), a success rate comparable to that achieved in treating breast cancer patients with either ablative or additive forms of endocrine therapy (12).

Though progestational therapy has been employed for the past quarter of a century, little is known concerning the mode of action of progestagens on primary and disseminated endometrial carcinoma. However, most investigators favor the notion that progestagens act directly on responsive endometrial carcinoma cells in much the same way as progesterone does on the endometrium of the menstrual cycle. During the postovulatory phase of the cycle progesterone transforms the estrogen-stimulated, proliferative endometrium to a secretory endometrium; that is, progesterone converts an actively growing and developing tissue to one that is more highly differentiated and essentially non-dividing. In clinical situations where progestagen treatment extends over several weeks or months, the endometrium may initially undergo differentiation but eventually becomes refractory and degenerates to a tissue having atrophic glands and sparse stroma. In general then, progestagens acting for relatively short durations

*No standard set of criteria has been adopted for objective remission of endometrial carcinoma. Therefore, the estimate of 30-35% remission must be considered in this light.

at physiological levels stimulate differentiation and inhibit mitosis, whereas progestagens acting over extended periods at pharmacological levels lead to marked suppression of the endometrium. These facets of progestagen action are thought to be the basis for the therapeutic effects of progestagens on endometrial carcinoma.

PROGESTATIONAL THERAPY OF ENDOMETRIAL CARCINOMA

Since this chapter is principally devoted to the mode of action of progestagens on endometrial carcinoma at the cellular and molecular level, progestational therapy *per se* will not be discussed. The interested reader is referred to the recent symposium volume, *Endometrial Cancer* edited by M.G. Brush, R.W. Taylor, and D.C. Williams, 1973 (10) and the American Cancer Society Conference, *New Directions for Research on Endometrial Cancer*, 1973 (11).

IN VITRO ACTION OF PROGESTAGENS

Several investigators have employed either short-term incubations or organ and cell culture systems to study the direct action of progestagens on human endometrium or endometrial carcinoma. Organ cultures of human endometrium show morphological and biochemical responses to progestagens that are comparable to those of the endometrium of the menstrual cycle (13), while the progestational response of endometrial carcinoma *in vitro* is similar to that seen following instillation of progesterone directly into the uterine cavity (7,14-17).

Early attempts to demonstrate progestational effects on the endometrium *in vitro* were not very successful. Ehrmann et al (18) who maintained human endometrium in organ culture found that the tissue explants passed through a secretory phase, independent of added estrogen and progesterone. Similarly, Figge (19) was unable to show any morphological or histochemical changes in human endometrium in either tissue or organ culture following estrogen or progesterone addition. Fortunately these early unrewarding attempts did not deter other investigators. Csermely et al (20,21) and Hughes et al (22,23) employing organ cultures of human endometrium, found that progesterone and synthetic progestagens induced histological, histochemical and biochemical changes similar to those observed during the secretory phase of the cycle. Control cultures retained a histological and biochemical pattern commensurate with the day of the cycle from which the specimens were taken. Following a 2-3 day exposure to progesterone (0.1 - 5 μg/ml) the endometrial glands increased in size, the epithelial cells became more columnar, the nuclei moved toward the lumen, and the secretory subnuclear vacuoles appeared. Glycogen deposition and alkaline phosphatase activity increased, followed by secretion of glycogen and alkaline phosphatase into the lumen. In contradistinction, when the progesterone concentration was raised to 10-50 μg/ml glandular development was suppressed. Kohorn and Tchao (24) maintained proliferative endometrial tissue in organ culture for 2-5 days. After two days of culture in the presence of 10μg of progesterone per ml, subnuclear vacuolation was observed in the glandular cells. By day 4 the subnuclear vacuoles had diminished and the histological appearance corresponded to that of a secretory endometrium, that is, the glandular cells were columnar and mucopolysaccharides were secreted into the lumen. The secretory changes brought on by this concentration of progesterone were not seen at higher concentrations of the hormone. At 50μg/ml, progesterone was clearly toxic, both glandular and stromal cells showing considerable necrosis.

Acute exposure of normal endometria to high concentrations of progesterone also inhibited nucleic acid synthesis. Nordqvist (25) incubated suspensions of curettage specimens from different days of the cycle with 0.8, 8 and 80 μg of progesterone per ml; labelled thymidine and uridine were used to measure rates of DNA and RNA synthesis, respectively. Progesterone at 8 and 80 μg/ml significantly inhibited RNA synthesis and 80 μg/ml inhibited DNA synthesis. Progesterone exerted its greatest inhibitory influence on DNA synthesis in specimens taken from the proliferative phase of the cycle, whereas the magnitude of RNA synthesis inhibition did not vary through the cycle. Since progesterone concentrations as high as 40-50 μg/ml are known to induce cellular necrosis, it seems likely that a portion of the diminished nucleic acid synthesis could be due to cytotoxicity.

In addition to the *in vitro* studies of normal endometria, Nordqvist (26-28), Kohorn and Tchao (29), Hustin (30) and Gerulath (31) have found that progesterone decreases nucleic acid synthesis and cell survival in a dose-dependent manner in endometrial carcinoma. Although the rate of nucleic acid synthesis varied considerably from carcinoma to carcinoma, DNA synthesis was consistently higher in poorly differentiated neoplasms. Noteworthy was the finding that 17β-estradiol potentiated the inhibitory action of progesterone on cell survival, particularly in poorly differentiated carcinomas. In ancillary studies Nordqvist (32) analyzed RNA and DNA synthesis in curettage specimens obtained from 12 patients before and after estrogen-progestagen therapy. Initially all 12 patients were given a single injection of 80 mg of polyestradiol phosphate and subsequently nine received 1250 mg of 17α-hydroxyprogesterone caproate twice weekly and three received 300 mg of 19-nor-17α-hydroxyprogesterone caproate twice weekly for periods of 3-7 weeks. Significant inhibition of DNA synthesis occurred in 10 cases, while RNA synthesis was markedly inhibited in all 12 patients. Since the *in vitro* effects of progesterone were also determined in the curettage specimens taken before *in vivo* estrogen-progestagen treatment, the response of individual carcinomas to progesterone *in vitro* and to estrogen-progestagens *in vivo* was compared. It was found that the relative response of DNA and RNA synthesis *in vitro* and *in vivo* was highly correlated (correlation coefficient = 0.90). Heckmann (33) also demonstrated that 19-nor-17α-hydroxyprogesterone caproate exerted marked cytostatic effects in primary cultures of adenocarcinoma.

Recently, Hiratsu (34) and Kuramoto and his colleagues (35,36) have reported the establishment of cell lines of human endometrium and endometrial adenocarcinoma which retain their original histological and cytogenic characteristics and respond to progestagens with a decrease in DNA synthesis and cell proliferation. These encouraging developments suggest that established human endometrial and adenocarcinoma cell lines may soon provide convenient model systems for studying the mechanism of action of progestagens.

PROGESTAGEN RECEPTORS

According to the hypothesis of a unitary mechanism of hormone action, hormone binding to target tissue receptors represents the primary event in the action of a hormone and as such is essential for the sequence of events or changes collectively referred to as the hormone response. If this hypothesis be correct, it follows that normal endometria and some endometrial carcinomas possess progestagen receptors that permit them to respond to progestagens. Indeed, progestagen receptors have now been detected in normal endometria (37-46) and in hyperplastic and carcinomatous endometria (40,41). By analogy to the known relationship between estrogen receptors and the response of breast cancer to endocrine therapies (12), the latter observation suggests that progestagen receptors might have prognostic value in deciding which endometrial cancer patients would respond to progestational therapy.

In 1971 Wiest and Rao (37) and Haukkamaa et al (40,41) demonstrated the existence of progesterone-specific binding proteins in normal endometria from uteri of hysterectomized patients. As reported at that time by Haukkamaa and coworkers (40,41) and subsequently by Bayard et al (46) binding activity was present throughout the cycle, but was highest during the late proliferative phase. This observation, along with the fact that administered estrogens induced progesterone receptors in the chick oviduct (47,48) and the guinea pig (49) and rabbit uterus (37), suggested that estrogens might be responsible for the elevated levels of progesterone receptor in the proliferative endometrium. More recently estrogen-priming has been found to induce progesterone receptors in the human (50), sheep (51,52), rat (53-55), mouse (53,54), and hamster (56,57) uterus. In contradistinction, the diminished levels of progesterone receptor during the secretory phase of the cycle (46) may be the result of negative control by progesterone. On the day of estrus in the hamster (56) and guinea pig (58,59) the concentration of progesterone-binding sites begins to fall at a time corresponding to preovulatory progesterone secretion and reaches a nadir during diestrus. Low levels of uterine progesterone receptor also have been noted during pregnancy in the rat (60) and guinea pig (58). Moreover, progesterone treatment of hamsters (56) and guinea pigs (61-64) causes a rapid depletion or inactivation of estrogen-induced progesterone receptors. Thus, the progesterone receptor concentration of the uterus is under dual hormonal control; 17β-estradiol exerts a positive control, i.e., it increases the concentration of receptor, whereas progesterone exerts a negative control, i.e., it lowers receptor levels. Negative control of progesterone receptor levels may explain why the endometrium becomes refractory and atrophic upon prolonged exposure to progestagens and, in addition, may have important implications with respect to the treatment of endometrial carcinoma with progestagens.

In addition to being estrogen-inducible, human uterine progesterone receptors (37-39,43-45,50) have been found to share many physicochemical properties in common with chick oviduct and other mammalian uterine receptors. These physicochemical properties are summarized as follows: 1) sedimentation coefficients of 3.7-4S and 7-8S, 2) equilibrium association constant of 1-4 x $10^9 M^{-1}$, 3) acidic proteins with isoelectric points of pH 4.8 and 5.2, 4) precipitated by 35% fractional saturation with $(NH_4)_2SO_4$, 5) heat labile, 6) stabilized by glycerol and sulfhydryl group protecting agents, and 7) sulfhydryl groups involved in binding. Smith et al (65) have recently achieved an 8000-fold purification of the 3.7S form of the receptor using a combination of $(NH_4)_2SO_4$ fractionation, affinity chromatography, and ion-exchange chromatography. The purified 3.7S protein migrated as a single band of molecular weight 110,000 on SDS polyacrylamide gel electrophoresis. This 3.7S protein also appeared to be the nuclear form of the receptor.

The steroid binding specificity of human endometrial and myometrial progesterone receptors has been extensively characterized and compared. Both receptor proteins displayed high specificity for progestagens (37-39,50,66,67) and had a correlation coefficient of 0.85 when ligands with a relative affinity value of greater than 1 (relative affinity for progesterone = 100) were compared (50). When the _in vitro_ binding affinities of the endometrial and myometrial receptors towards progestagens were compared with the _in vivo_ biological activities of the same steroids, a fairly good correlation was seen in most instances (38,39,50,66,67). Where significant disagreement occurred it was usually possible to explain this on the basis of _in vivo_ metabolic transformation and/or half-life.

Very few data are available concerning the existence of progesterone receptors in hyperplastic and carcinomatous endometria. Using equilibrium dialysis Haukkamaa and colleagues (40,41) examined seven specimens of simple hyperplasia, two of adenomatous hyperplasia, six of endometrial carcinoma, and five of atrophic endometrium. Simple hyperplastic endometria showed variable progesterone binding capacity which was comparable to that of normal endometria. The two specimens of adenomatous hyperplasia and four out of six specimens of endometrial carcinoma also showed varying degrees of specific progesterone binding. The two remaining endometrial carcinomas and all five cases of atrophic endometrium lacked progesterone binders. Rao et al (38) and Young and Cleary (45) each examined two carcinomatous endometria but were unable to detect progesterone receptors in any of the neoplasms. Based on these fragmentary data, one might postulate that if endometrial hyperplasia is an intermediate in the pathway leading to neoplasia, then the loss of progesterone receptors occurs at a step beyond this point. In support, most endometrial hyperplasias or dysplasias are reversible when normal menstrual cycles are established or when progestagen therapy is employed (68,69). Four out of 10 carcinomas contained progesterone binding proteins, a fraction approximating the remission rate following progestational therapy.

Though progestagen receptors are necessary, they may not be sufficient for hormone-induced remission. This caveat may be illustrated by the recent work of McGuire (70) which shows that only 55-60% of breast tumors with estrogen receptors respond to hormonal manipulation. McGuire postulated that a biochemical lesion may occur at a later step in hormone action, thereby rendering the tissue unresponsive to endocrine therapy. McGuire's initial data using the progesterone receptor as a marker for estrogen responsiveness provide considerable support for his hypothesis. In addition, there is some indication in endometrial carcinomas that the response to progestagen therapy is better in those patients who have recently been subjected to estrogens (71,72). One possible explanation is that estrogen-priming induces progestagen receptors that permit the carcinoma to respond to progestational therapy. Moreover, it is known that premenopausal women respond more frequently to progestational therapy than do postmenopausal women (73).

Because of the strong possibility that estrogen and progestagen receptors may determine whether endocrine therapy of endometrial carcinoma will be successful, it would appear highly desirable to establish a multi-center screening program to correlate the presence of receptors with hormone responsiveness. The Breast Cancer Task Force Program might serve well as a useful prototype for this type of screening effort.

REFERENCES

1. Kelley, R.M. and W.H. Baker, In: Pincus, G. and E.P. Vollmer (eds.), Biological Activities of Steroids in Relation to Cancer, Academic Press, New York, 1960, p. 427.

2. Kistner, R.W., Cancer 12:1106, 1959.

3. Varga, A. and E. Henriksen, Obstet. Gynecol. 18:658, 1961.

4. Stoll, B.A., Cancer Chemother. Rep. 14:83, 1961.

5. Jolles, B., Brit. J. Cancer 16:209, 1962.

6. Kennedy, B.J.A., J. Amer. Med. Assoc. 184:758, 1963.

7. Wentz, W.B., Obstet. Gynecol. 24:370, 1964.

8. Bergsjo, P., Acta Endocrinol. 59:412, 1965.

9. Frick, H.C., II, Metabolism 14:348, 1965.

10. Brush, M.G., R.W. Taylor and D.C. Williams (eds.), Endometrial Cancer, William Heinemann Medical Books Ltd., London, 1973.

11. New Directions for Research on Endometrial Cancer. Gynecol. Oncology 2:113, 1974.

12. McGuire, W.L., P.P. Carbone and E.P. Vollmer (eds.), Estrogen Receptors in Human Breast Cancer, Raven Press, New York, 1975.

13. Lawn, A.M., In: Bishop, M.W.H. (ed.), Advances in Reproductive Physiology, Vol. 6, Elek Science, Ltd., London, 1973, p. 61.

14. Truskett, I.D., In: Shearman, R.P. (ed.), Recent Advances in Ovarian and Synthetic Steroids, Sydney, Australia, 1964, p. 140.

15. Kistner, R.W., C.T. Griffiths and J.M. Craig, Cancer 18: 1563, 1965.

16. Hustin, J., J. Obstet. Gynaecol. Br. Commonw. 77:915, 1970.

17. Hustin, J., In: Brush, M.G., R.W. Taylor and D.C. Williams (eds.), Endometrial Cancer, William Heinemann Medical Books, Ltd., London, 1973, p. 246.

18. Ehrmann, R.L., H.A. McKelvey and A.T. Hertig, Obstet. Gynecol. 17:416, 1961.

19. Figge, D.C., Acta Cytol. 7:245, 1963.

20. Csermely, T., L.M. Demers and E.C. Hughes, Obstet. Gynecol. 34:252, 1969.

21. Csermely, T., E.C. Hughes and L.M. Demers, Am. J. Obstet. Gynec. 109:1066, 1971.

22. Hughes, E.C., L.M. Demers, T. Csermely and D.B. Jones, Am. J. Obstet. Gynec. 105:707, 1969.

23. Hughes, E.C., T. Csermely, R.D. Jacobs and P.A. O'Hern, Gynecol. Oncology 2:205, 1974.

24. Kohorn, E.I. and R. Tchao, J. Endocrinol. 45:401, 1969.

25. Nordqvist, S., J. Endocrinol. 48:17, 1970.

26. Nordqvist, S., J. Endocrinol. 48:29, 1970.

27. Nordqvist, S., Acta Obstet. Gynecol. Scand. 49:275, 1970.

28. Nordqvist, S., Acta Obstet. Gynecol. Scand. Suppl. 19:25, 1971.

29. Kohorn, E.I. and M. Chir, J. Obstet. Gynaecol. Br. Commonw. 75:1262, 1968.

30. Hustin, J., Br. J. Obstet. Gynaecol. 82:493, 1975.

31. Gerulath, A.H., Clin. Res. 23:643A, 1975.

32. Nordqvist, S., In: Brush, M.G., R.W. Taylor and D.C. Williams (eds.), Endometrial Cancer, William Heinemann Medical Books, Ltd., London, 1973, p. 33.

33. Heckmann, U., Ger. Med. Mon. 11:48, 1966.

34. Hiratsu, T., Kobe J. Med. Sci. 14:29, 1968.

35. Kuramoto, H., S. Tamura and Y. Notake, Am. J. Obstet. Gynec. 114:1012, 1972.

36. Kuramoto, H., Acta Obstet. Gynaecol. Japon. 19:47, 1972.

37. Wiest, W.G. and B.R. Rao, In: Raspe, G. (ed.), Advances in the Biosciences, Vol. 7, Pergamon Press, Vieweg, New York, 1971, p. 251.

38. Rao, B.R., W.G. Wiest and W.M. Allen, Endocrinology 95:1275, 1975.

39. Rao, B.R. and W.G. Wiest, Gynecol. Oncology 2:239, 1974.

40. Haukkamaa, M., O. Karjalainen and T. Luukkainen, Am. J. Obstet. Gynec. 111:205, 1971.

41. Haukkamaa, M., O. Karjalainen and T. Luukkainen, J. Steroid Biochem. 3:631, 1972.

42. Haukkamaa, M. and T. Luukkainen, J. Steroid Biochem. 5:447, 1974.

43. Crocker, S.G., J.R. Thompson and R.J.B. King, Acta Endocrinol. Suppl. 177:244, 1973.

44. Philbert, D. and J.P. Raynaud, Contraception 10:457, 1974.

45. Young, P.C. and R.E. Clearly, J. Clin. Endocrinol. Metab. 39:425, 1974.

46. Bayard, F., S. Damilano, P. Robel and E.-E. Baulieu, C.R. Acad. Sci. Paris Series D 281:1341, 1975.

47. O'Malley, B.W., M.R. Sherman and D.O. Toft, Proc. Natl. Acad. Sci., U.S.A. 67:501, 1970.

48. O'Malley, B.W., M.R. Sherman, D.O. Toft, T.C. Spelsberg, W.T. Schader and A.W. Steggles, In: Raspe, G. (ed.), Advances in the Biosciences, Vol. 7, Pergamon Press, Vieweg, New York, 1971, p. 213.

49. Milgrom, E., M. Atger and E.-E. Baulieu, In: Raspe, G. (ed.), Advances in the Biosciences, Vol. 7, Pergamon Press, Vieweg, New York, 1971, p. 235.

50. Jänne, O., T. Kontula, T. Luukkainen and R. Vihko, J. Steroid Biochem. 6:501, 1975.

51. Kontula, K., O. Jänne, E. Rajakowki, E. Tanhuanpaa and R. Vihko, J. Steroid Biochem. 5:39, 1974.

52. Kontula, K., Acta Endocrinol. 78:593, 1975.

53. Feil, P.D., S.R. Glasser, D.O. Toft and B.W. O'Malley, Endocrinology 91:738, 1972.

54. Philibert, D. and J.-P. Raynaud, Steroids 22:89, 1973.

55. Faber, L.E., M.L. Sandmann and H.E. Stavely, J. Biol. Chem. 247:5648, 1972.

56. Leavitt, W.W., D.O. Toft, C.A. Strott and B.W. O'Malley, Endocrinology 94:1041, 1974.

57. Reel, J.R. and Y. Shih, Acta Endocrinol. 80:344, 1975.

58. Milgrom, E., M. Atger, M. Perrot and E.-E. Baulieu, Endocrinology 90:1071, 1972.

59. Milgrom, E., M. Luu Thi and E.-E. Baulieu, Acta Endocrinol. Suppl. 180:380, 1973.

60. Davies, I.J. and K.J. Ryan, Endocrinology 92:394, 1973.

61. Milgrom, E., M. Luu Thi, M. Atger and E.-E. Baulieu, J. Biol. Chem. 248:6366, 1973.

62. Luu Thi, M. and E. Milgrom, C.R. Acad. Sci. Paris Series D 276:2281, 1973.

63. Freifeld, M.L., P.D. Feil and C.W. Bardin, Steroids 23: 93, 1974.

64. Luu Thi, M., E.-E. Baulieu and E. Milgrom, J. Endocrinol. 66:349, 1975.

65. Smith, R.G., C.A. Iramain, V.C. Buttram and B.W. O'Malley, Nature 253:271, 1975.

66. Kontula, K., O. Jänne, R. Vihko, E. deJager, J. deVisser and F. Zeelen, Acta Endocrinol. 78:574, 1975.

67. Smith, H.E., R.G. Smith, D.O. Toft, J.R. Neergaard, E.P. Burrows and B.W. O'Malley, J. Biol. Chem. 249:5924, 1974.

68. Vellios, F., Gynecol. Oncology 2:152, 1974.

69. Wentz, W.B., Gynecol. Oncology 2:362, 1974.

70. McGuire, W.L., In: Menon, K.M.J. and J.R. Reel (eds.), Steroid Hormone Action and Cancer, Plenum Press, New York, 1976, p. 28.

71. Sherman, A.I., Obstet. Gynecol. 28:309, 1966.

72. Smith, J.P., F. Rutledge and S.W. Soffar, Am. J. Obstet. Gynec. 94:977, 1966.

73. Carbone, P.P. and S.K. Carter, Gynecol. Oncology 2:348, 1974.

ARE ORAL CONTRACEPTIVES AND DIETHYLSTILBESTROL (DES) INVOLVED IN SEX-LINKED CANCER?[a]

Richard A. Edgren

Department of Pharmacology
Parke, Davis and Company
Ann Arbor, Michigan

A roundtable discussion on this subject was held on the afternoon of October 28, 1975. In addition to me as Chairman, panelists were: Roy Hertz, M.D., Research Professor, Department of Pharmacology, The George Washington University Medical Center, Washington, D.C. and Frank M. Sturtevant, Ph.D., Associate Director, Research and Development, Searle Laboratories, G.D. Searle and Company, Chicago, Illinois.

In an effort to deal with the broad implications of this area the two subjects have been separated, since 1) DES is not steroidal, as opposed to the estrogens in the oral contraceptives, and 2) the pattern of administration differs between the two types of compounds. In each of the sections, introductory statements were made by the chairman and then discussed first by the panelists and then from the floor.

ORAL CONTRACEPTIVES

Effect of Oral Contraceptives and Their Components in Laboratory Animals

Since oral contraceptives are combinations of estrogens and progestagens given together or are progestagens administered alone (minipills), one must examine the effects of the compounds indepen-

[a]See Comments section for notes indicated by superscript letters.

dently and their combinations in order to gain any firm understanding of the effects of these drugs.

Estrogens. Since the estrogens have been examined extensively and intensively, they are a satisfactory point of departure. Only two estrogens are employed as components of oral contraceptives: ethinyl estradiol (EE) and its 3-methyl ether, mestranol. Neither has been employed in rodents for cancer studies for as long as diethylstilbestrol or natural estrogens, but both have had extensive examination as aspects of safety studies on oral contraceptives. The "Scowen Committee" report (1) summarizes rodent experiments. Large numbers of benign pituitary tumors were seen in both sexes, and in most studies in mice. Inspection of the data suggests that EE was more effective than mestranol. In rats, mestranol and estrone were associated with increased incidences of tumors in females in one, but not in three other studies. Gonadal tumors, all benign, tended to be of no significance in most studies, although in rats, one study showed a slight excess of tumors with EE. Two studies on mice, using a Swiss Random strain or BDH-SPF (Carshalton stock) had increased incidences of gonadal tumors in both sexes with both estrogens. The females of the latter strain also had high incidences of malignant tumors of the uterus (fundus and cervix) on EE, whereas other groups did not. Finally, an increased incidence of malignant mammary tumors was seen with these two sensitive strains of mice, and in female rats treated with EE, mestranol or estrone.

Few studies with estrogens alone have been carried out with dogs, but no major increase either in benign or malignant lesions appears to occur. (See review by Drill and associates, 2,3,4,5). Similarly, the Rhesus monkeys seem not to show increased incidence of carcinoma in response to estrogens (2,3,4,5).

Dr. Hertz pointed out that the development of mammary tumors is accelerated by hormone exposure. In dogs, Jabara (6) has seen mesotheliomatous tumors of the ovary that are malignant, invasive and metastasizing with stilbestrol. These are not affected by simultaneous progesterone administration.[b] Rhesus monkeys show no tumors in response to estrogens, but McClure (7) showed that stilbestrol produced malignant mesotheliomas in squirrel monkey uterine walls and throughout the abdominal and pleural cavities, suggesting that the species of primate employed is critically important. Dr. Edgren asked Dr. Hertz about the dose levels used, pointing out that rodent studies carried out during the 1930's and 1940's used massive amounts of estrogens. Dr. Hertz admitted that the doses used were very large and that good dose-response relationships did not exist. In both the squirrel monkeys and dogs, the estrogen used was DES, and not one of the components of oral contraceptives.

Dr. Sturtevant added that Rudali and associates (8) had recently published on the tumorigenic effects of estriol pellets in mice.

Progestagens have rarely been associated with the kind of tumorigenesis shown by the estrogens in rodents, although the Scowen Committee report showed high incidences of pituitary tumors in mice that received norethynodrel and norethisterone (norethindrone). No marked increase in gonadal tumors was reported and mammary and uterine tissues were apparently unaffected quantitatively. In rats, norethynodrel was associated with a marked increase in pituitary tumors in males and a decrease in females. None of the other progestagens induced obvious increases in benign pituitary tumors. Meaningful increases in gonadal tumors were not apparent. Increases in benign mammary tumors following norethynodrel, norethindrone and ethynodiol diacetate in males were counterbalanced by decreased incidence in females; these three compounds were also associated with increases in malignant tumors in both sexes, whereas slight increases were seen with chlormadinone acetate, lynestrenol and megestrol acetate in females.

Over the past several years, the development of mammary tumors in dogs under treatment with progestagens has occasioned close attention, including the withdrawal of chlormadinone acetate from the market, and the termination of clinical trials with various chloroethynyl derivatives and relatives of 19-nortestosterone and megestrol acetate. These lesions are reported to be characteristically benign and their development appears to be accelerated by the progestagens (2,3,5,0); early data did not show that the incidence was grossly increased over control levels (10).

Rhesus monkey data seem largely restricted to estrogens alone and combinations.

Dr. Hertz pointed out that Lipschutz and associates (11) produced no ovarian tumors with norethindrone after about 1-2 years of exposure, but that at autopsy a year later tumors were apparent.[c] In dogs, Hertz stated that approximately 10% of tumors in beagles show areas of highly invasive carcinomas (11a).[d]

Sturtevant stated that in mice genetic differences among strains and susceptibility to viruses make data extremely difficult to interpret. Two of the progestagens implicated in dog tumorigenesis, chlormadinone acetate and megestrol acetate, have considerable glucocorticoid activity, which may be of significance.

Combinations. Again, the Scowen Committee report seems germane to a discussion of the rodent data. Their conclusions (1) point out that mammary and pituitary tumors follow the pattern of effects expected from the estrogen literature, i.e., increased incidences in susceptible strains at high doses and when materials are administered over a major portion of the life span. Further, these effects seem to be largely conditioned by the estrogenic component.

The dog studies have focused heavily on the effects of the progestagen, however, the combinations appear to have somewhat similar effects (2,3,5,10). Rhesus monkeys seem not to develop tumors in response to oral contraceptives (4,11a)[e], although a single oral contraceptive-treated animal died from an infiltrating ductal carcinoma of the breast and metastases (12).

Currently neither the dog nor the monkey studies appear to suggest an immediate danger.

Effect of Oral Contraceptives in Humans

So far the most definitive statement appears to be that of the Royal College of General Practitioners (13). This report concludes (p.22): "There is no evidence that the Pill increases the risk of malignancy. A protective effect of oral contraceptives on the occurrence of benign breast neoplasia is confirmed." Drill (2, 3,5) and Taber (14) have reviewed current data, both retrospective and prospective, on breast cancer without uncovering evidence of increased incidence in women taking oral contraceptives.

Sturtevant questioned the quotation from the Royal College Report on benign breast disease, since the studies presumably confirmed were retrospective; since retrospective studies cannot provide a basis for scientific proof of causation, a prospective study cannot confirm this "proof".

Both Sturtevant and Hertz pointed out that the time period was too short for definitive conclusions and Hertz read into the record the following statement from p.25 of the Royal College report: "....The evidence concerning a possible carcinogenic effect of the Pill is so far reassuring. It must be emphasized, however, that observations are required on a large number of women who have used the Pill for a minimum of ten years before any confident conclusions can be drawn."[f]

Questions from the Floor

1) Are British and American data applicable to other countries and races?

The Panel agreed that these were the best available data and could only apply directly to the populations in question. Similar data will have to be drawn for other races before equivalent conclusions will be possible.

2) Since pregnancy affects incidence and rates of development of breast cancer would the oral contraceptive have similar effects?

Dr. Hertz pointed out the extreme complexity of this question. Early use of OC's will delay first term pregnancies to an increased age and thus increase breast cancer likelihood; the OC's themselves only poorly simulate endocrine changes in pregnancy, i.e., adrenal changes, endocrinology of the fetal-placental unit, etc., and therefore a pregnancy effect on cancer is unlikely to relate directly to the effects of OC's.

3) In response to a question on some early reports of a protective effect of OC's on cervical cancer Hertz discussed unpublished data from the Communicable Disease Center purporting to show a more frequent and rapid progression of Papanicolaou smears from dysplasia to carcinoma-in-situ in OC than in control patients. To date definitive statements cannot be made.

Summary

To date, information on oral contraceptives provides us with no evidence of the induction of human carcinoma with the use of these drugs. However, animal studies do suggest some possible concern and demand close surveillance.

DIETHYLSTILBESTROL (DES)

Threatened Abortion and Other Pregnancy Problems

Historically, during the 1940's the Smiths (and others) recommended the use of DES in a broad range of pregnancy problems. The Smiths (15) believed that DES somehow increased the ovarian production of progesterone which was effective in salvaging the pregnancy. With time, estrogens came most commonly to be employed in threatened and habitual abortion and maternal diabetes. Serious doubts were soon expressed concerning the efficacy of such treatment, leading to one of the earliest double-blind, placebo-controlled clinical studies, that of the Chicago Lying-In Hospital group (16). (The excellent Ferguson study, which antedates the Chicago paper, only misses modern criteria of excellence by not being double-blind, 16a). Their conclusion was that DES had no therapeutic value. However, the dramatic hemostatic effect of DES and other estrogens supported continued use for spotting during early pregnancy. Like many therapeutic modalities of questionable efficacy, DES in threatened and habitual abortion seemed destined for footnote status in medical histories (Eli Lilly removed the "indication" in 1967) until 1971 when Herbst, Ulfelder and Poskanzer (17) reported eight cases of vaginal carcinoma in young women, seven of whom had been delivered by mothers after DES treatment during pregnancy. In a characteristic retrospective study, these patients were compared with a series of "controls", none of whom had DES in their history, and a magnificent P-value was obtained with an unnecessarily sophisticated chi-square test. Subsequently, a large number of additional patients have come to light, including a significant proportion who have no history of maternal therapy (18), and thus demonstrate the inappropriate nature of the original control group. Despite the weakness of their data, Herbst and associates (18) estimate that the frequency of carcinoma in exposed girls is "...much less..." than the estimate of the Mayo Clinic group (19) which itself was "...less than 4 per 1000...". This latter figure is of particular interest since it was based on an academic exercise in a retrospective study in which "No adenocarcinoma of the vagina or cervix was found..." in 818 females whose mothers had received estrogens during pregnancy (93% of the mothers had received DES). Unfortunately, the caveat that introduces this exercise: "Assuming a true association exists between <u>in utero</u> exposure to synthetic estrogens and clear-cell adenocarcinoma of the vagina and cervix in young women, we have attempted to define the risk of developing this type of cancer after such exposure", is likely to become separated in both the literature and the mind. If a causal relationship exists this extremely low estimated incidence of carcinoma may explain the fact that "...no case of adenocarcinoma of the vagina or cervix occurring in a young woman exposed to oestrogens <u>in utero</u> has yet been reported in the United Kingdom" and a follow-up of the Chicago Lying-In Hospital double-blind study has failed to uncover a case in 84 DES-exposed females (20).[g] Of the cancers about 30-40% are cervical and the remainder vaginal.

In contradistinction to cancer, vaginal adenosis seems likely to be induced by DES, as shown by the Chicago follow-up (20). However, the relationship between adenosis and carcinoma remains unclear. Ulfelder (21) has noted the absence of demonstrated progression from adenosis to carcinoma; further 8-10% of the cancers are not associated with adenosis. Stafl and Mattingly (22) provide a scheme allowing for such a progression.

The relationship between DES and human vaginal cancers is certainly not clear and the discussion pointed out differences in opinion among the panelists. Dr. Hertz seemed willing to accept available retrospective data as proof of a causal relationship, whereas both Edgren and Sturtevant took the position that the case was not proved and basically not provable from such studies. If a causal relationship actually exists, Edgren expressed a willingness to accept the retrospective studies as descriptive. Obviously, should an adenosis-carcinoma progression be established further follow-up of the Chicago Lying-In Hospital double-blind study will be crucial. In any event, even should a clear causality be established, current data suggest that it will not be a simple one of classical carcinogenesis. Hertz (21) has called this type of response a teratocarcinogenic effect. Stafl and Mattingly (22) have stated:

> The biological effect of DES is one of teratogenesis, rather than carcinogenesis, and induces congenital alterations in the vaginal extension of columnar epithelium where the possibility of neoplastic transformation can occur at a later age through a mutagenic agent other than DES.

Questions from the floor involved the efficacy of DES therapy in problem pregnancies. Both Edgren and Sturtevant appeared willing to reject this form of therapy as probably useless, while Hertz was unwilling to deny its utility completely.

As Post-Coital Contraceptive

The administration of large doses of estrogen to women shortly after unprotected, isolated coitus is followed by an extremely low incidence of pregnancy, suggesting an effect of the estrogen in preventing some aspect of early gestation (23,24,25,26). Controlled studies have not been carried out, but there would seem to be little doubt of the efficacy of DES (23,24,26) while lesser data on EE (24,25) and other estrogens are suggestive.

The mode-of-action of the estrogens is not well established. Edgren cited the similarity between this human use and the tubal effects in animals (low dose acceleration of egg transport and high dose inhibition, tubal lock, in some species). In contradistinction, Dr. Hertz insisted that the anti-fertility effect in humans resulted from biochemical changes in the endometrium that precluded nidation. The review of Blye (25) mentions both possibilities, as well as others.

The possible danger of this type of therapy, at least with respect to cancer, was disposed of rapidly by the panel. The post-coital use of estrogens, and particularly DES, is high-dose, short-term therapy, quite different from the high-dose, long-term approach usually associated with carcinogenesis. Therefore, danger to the woman taking an estrogen correctly[h] would seem minimal. Further, danger for the fetus seems of little significance, even if DES is conclusively proved to be carcinogenic. If pregnancy is prevented, no danger can exist; however, later abortion should be recommended in the event of an unsuccessful termination.

Questions from the Floor

Questions from the floor involved possible evidence of a carcinogenic effect of estrogens in humans receiving long-term therapy for prostatic or mammary carcinoma. Dr. Hertz pointed out that most such therapy was employed in advanced prostatic carcinoma and too few patients survived for long enough periods to give critical information. In the female with breast cancer, massive doses of DES have been given for 1-3 years. Studies of the development of cancer in the contralateral breast do not show increases over the 6% seen in the untreated population.[i]

No carcinogenic effects of phytoestrogens were known to members of the panel.

Duration and dosage problems with DES were discussed. Data on dose and time do not suggest any clear dose-response or temporal relationship; with the latter point modified by the concept that treatment must cover the time of organogenesis and differentiation of the Müllerian duct system for adenosis. Further, a significant proportion of the cases have no known exposure to hormone therapy and males seem refractory.

COMMENTS

[a]This summary of the discussion has been prepared primarily from a tape recording of the proceedings; the inevitable and now expected gaps in this recording have been filled in from my manual notes of the meeting and from memory. The text has been sent to both Drs. Hertz and Sturtevant for review and their comments returned for incorporation in the text. I have, however, taken the editorial prerogative of deleting repetitive material discussed elsewhere in this volume and in the roundtable. Further, I have taken the liberty of commenting briefly in this section on some references, cited in passing during the discussion, that I have reviewed since. I have also expanded more extensively on sources of information that supported the initial, generalized statements than was possible in the oral presentation. The section on DES has been read by Dr. Jerry M. Maas of The Eli Lilly Company and Dr. John Gunning of Harbor General Hospital, Torrance, California. Both made valuable comments for

which I am indebted. Finally, as an opponent of the advocacy school of journalism, I have attempted honestly to cite the evidence selected by each of us in support of our often conflicting views and conclusions, and I trust that these conflicts will be evident from the text. Although I have attempted to be an objective reporter and editor, inevitably my own position will create biases, attitudes and emphases that may prove unacceptable to other panel members; responsibility for the text, therefore, is mine, exclusively (R.A.E.).

[b]In this uncontrolled study, all 13 animals treated developed tumors 3-14 months after injection of stilbestrol injections; 12 were invasive neoplasms and 9 were metastatic. Breed of dog varied, as did age, duration of experiment and dose.

[c]I find myself rather challenged to understand the experimental design employed in this study; the final interpretation is even more difficult to follow. The effects of norethindrone and norethynodrel appear to be controlled by studies on "normal" and progesterone-treated mice, although these were apparently not simultaneous controls, but came from other experiments done at other times; further, whether the "normal" animals had cholesterol pellets or not is unclear; steroid-treated mice were housed with males, nothing is said about controls, normal or progesterone, or pregnancies, if any, with any group. The authors conclude (Summary): "Ovarian granulosa cell tumors are elicited in mice by the prolonged administration of norethindrone and norethynodrel". Their data show (Table IV):

Treatment	N Mice	N with Tumors
Normal	33	1
Progesterone	44	1
Norethindrone	25	13
Norethynodrel	24	2

These numerical data certainly prove no statistically acceptable proof of a tumorigenic effect of either norethynodrel or progesterone.

[d]Review of the Finkel-Berliner paper shows statements concerning metastases with medroxyprogesterone acetate and anagestone, and invasiveness is attributed to chlormadinone acetate; the "approximately 10%" would seem to have another origin. Incidences of reported nodules increased with extended time over those used in previous analysis (10).

[e]That the monkeys (Rhesus) are "clean" is supported by the statement: "Although these studies have been conducted for a period over 5 years in some cases, the monkeys have demonstrated only a very occasional mammary nodule or local mammary hyperplasia..."(11a).

[f]Statements of this kind are occasioned by the relatively long human latent period of development of cancer following exposure to carcinogenic substances (see Hertz, this volume). It seems peculiar, however, that this latent period problem has not generated skepticism concerning the nature of the relationship between conjugated estrogens and uterine carcinoma recently inferred from retrospective studies. In one study (27) almost 2/3 of the exposed patients where data on duration were available had had less than 7 years of exposure; the second study (28) appears to ignore this factor, although the Methods include: "....estrogen treatment, with a record of at least six months of estrogen used before endometrial cancer was diagnosed....".

[g]Additional negative results in large series were reported by John Gunning at the recent North American Conference on Fertility and Sterility on January 30, 1976, Acapulco, Mexico. Townsend examined 600 DES exposures and Gunning over 200 with no cases of vaginal cancer.

[h]The lay press and Congressional witnesses have suggested a large amount of repetitive usage; in such circumstances the panel's opinion may be inapplicable.

[i]Here again the short duration of study must be considered in the light of the long human latent period for induction of carcinoma.

REFERENCES

1. Carcinogenicity tests of oral contraceptives. A report by The Committee on Safety of Medicines. Her Majesty's Stationery Office, London, 1972.

2. Drill, V.A., Excerpta Medica Internatl. Congr. Ser. 131: 192, 1973.

3. Drill, V.A., Ibid:200, 1973.

4. Drill, V.A., D.P. Martin, E.R. Hart and R.C. McConnell, J. Nat. Cancer Inst. 52:1655, 1974.

5. Drill, V.A., Ann. Rev. Pharmacology 15:367, 1962.

6. Jabara, A.O., Australian J. Exp. Biol. 40:130, 1962.

7. McClure, H.M. and C.E. Graham, Lab. Animal Sci. 232:493, 1973.

8. Rudali, G., F. Apiou and B. Meul, Europ. J. Cancer 11;39, 1975.

9. Nelson, L.W., J.H. Weikel, Jr. and F.E. Reno, J. Nat. Cancer Inst. 51:1303, 1973.

10. Edgren, R.A., Clin. Proc. Internatl. Planned Parenthood Fed. S.E. Asia & Oceania Regional Med. Sci. Congr., Sydney, p.144, 1973.

11. Lipschutz, A., R. Iglesias, V.I. Panasevich and S. Salinas, Brit. J. Cancer 31:153, 1967.

11a. Finkel, M.J. and V.R. Berliner, Bull. Soc. Pharmacol. & Path. 4:13, 1973.

12. Kirschstein, R.L., A.S. Robson and G.W. Reisten, J. Nat. Cancer Inst. 48:551, 1972.

13. Oral contraceptives and health - an interim report from the oral contraception study of the Royal College of General Practitioners. Pitman, London and New York, 1974.

14. Taber, B.A., J. Reprod. Med. 15:97, 1975.

15. Smith, O.W., G. van S. Smith and D. Hurwitz, Amer. J. Obstet. Gynec. 51:411, 1946.

16. Dieckmann, W.J., M.E. Davis, L.M. Rynkiewicz and R.E. Pottinger, Ibid 66:1062, 1953.

16a. Ferguson, J.H., Ibid. 65:592, 1953.

17. Herbst, A.L., H. Ulfelder and D.C. Poskanzer, New Engl. J. Med. 284:878, 1971.

18. Herbst, A.L., R.E. Scully and S.J. Robbay, J. Reprod. Med. 15:5, 1975.

19. Lanier, A.P., K.L. Noller and D.G. Decker, Mayo Clinic Proc. 48:793, 1973.

20. Bibbo, M., M. Al-Nafee, T. Baccarini, W. Gill, M. Newton, K.M. Sleeper, M. Sonek and G.L. Weed, J. Reprod. Med. 15: 29, 1975.

21. Hertz, R., In: Menon, K.M.J. and J.R. Reel (eds.), Steroid Hormone Action and Cancer, Plenum Press, New York, 1976, p.1.

22. Stafl, A. and R.F. Mattingly, Amer. J. Obstet. Gynec. 120: 666, 1974.

23. Kuchera, L.K., J. Amer. Med. Assn. 281:562, 1971.

24. Morris, J.M. and G. van Wagenen, Amer. J. Obstet. Gynec. 115:101, 1973.

25. Blye, R.P., Ibid. 116:1044, 1973.

26. Rosenfeld, D.L., G.R. Hoggins, A.M. Jusczyk, C.R. Garcia and K. Rickels, Medical, psychological and social factors in morning-after pill utilization. (Meeting Assn. Planned Parenthood Physicians, Los Angeles, April 17-18, 1975). Family Planning Perspectives 7:151, 1975.

27. Zeil, D.C. and W.D. Finkle, New Engl. J. Med. 293:1167, 1975.

28. Smith, D.C., R. Prentice, D.J. Thompson and W.L. Herrmann, Ibid.:1164, 1975.

RADIOIODINATED ESTROGENS AND ANTIESTROGENS AS POTENTIAL IMAGING AGENTS

R.E. Counsell, A. Buswink, N. Korn, M. Johnson,
V. Ranade, and T. Yu

Laboratory of Medicinal Chemistry, College of Pharmacy
University of Michigan, Ann Arbor, Michigan

In an earlier chapter, Dr. William McGuire reviewed studies demonstrating that estradiol is selectively taken up by certain mammary tumors in addition to other target tissues such as uterus and pituitary. It has been our goal for the past ten years to synthesize an agent labelled with a gamma-emitting nuclide that would mimic estradiol in this selective uptake process. Theoretically, such an agent would be a useful diagnostic agent in Nuclear Medicine for the imaging of estrogen responsive tissues and tumors.

The radionuclide we have chosen for our initial studies is radioiodine because of: a) its versatility in incorporation into organic molecules and b) its availability in several different, medically useful, isotopic forms. Iodine-125 has been employed in the present studies because its long half-life (60 days) and low radiation energy (35 KeV) simplify synthesis, storage, and animal experiments.

Thus, the procedure we have followed has been to:

1. synthesize an iodinated estrogen analog,
2. evaluate its ability to compete with estradiol in the estrogen receptor protein assay (in vitro),
3. evaluate its in vivo estrogenicity in the female immature mouse assay,
4. incorporate radioiodine by isotope exchange procedures into those compounds selected on the basis of the above tests, and
5. evaluate the tissue distribution of the radioiodinated estrogen in immature and mature female rats.

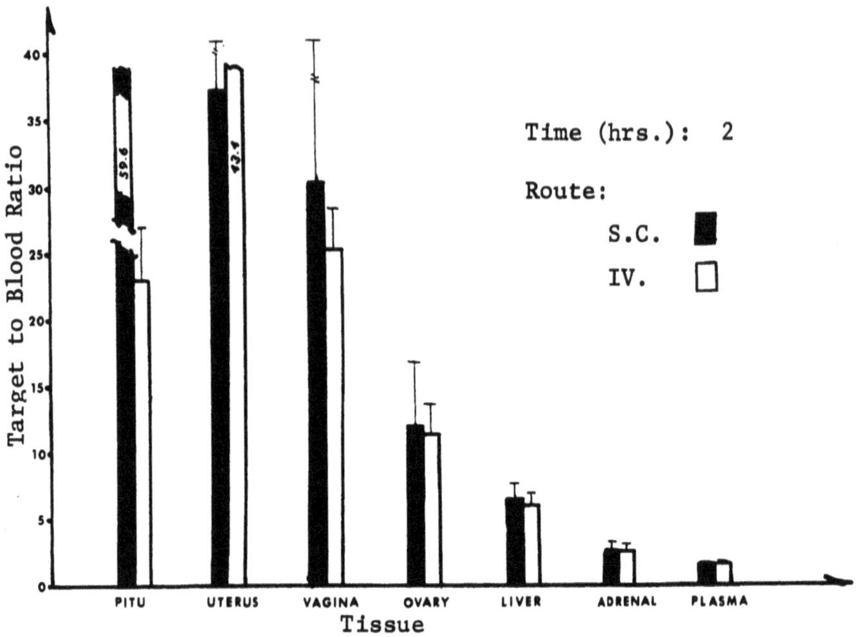

Fig 1. Target to Blood Ratios for Estradiol-17β (Sp. Act. = 176 mCi/mg) in Immature Sprague-Dawley Female Rats (± S.E.M.).

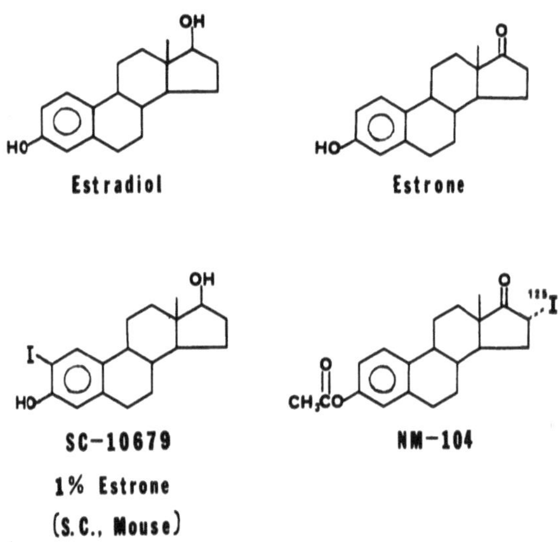

Fig 2. Steroidal Estrogens.

As noted by previous workers (1,2), the immature female rat is particularly well suited for estrogen tissue distribution studies. At this early stage of development, the receptor proteins are present in the target tissues but the endogenous circulating estrogen titer is low. Fig 1 illustrates the tissue distribution of estradiol-^{3}H in this animal model. Target tissues such as pituitary, uterus and vagina show tissue to blood ratios greater than 20. Results were similar for both intravenous and subcutaneous routes of administration.

In the early phases of our study, we focused on the natural steroid hormones (Fig 2) as the possible carriers for radioiodine. 2-Iodoestradiol (SC-10679) was synthesized by direct iodination, but was found to have only 1% the activity of estrone in the mouse uterus weight assay. Since _ortho_ iodinated phenols are known to deiodinate _in vivo_ (3), this modest estrogenic activity could have been the result of _in vivo_ conversion of 2-iodoestradiol to estradiol.

Similarly, 16-iodoestrone 3-acetate-^{125}I (NM-104) was synthesized according to a literature procedure (4) and radioiodine introduced by isotope exchange. As might be anticipated for an α-iodoketone, tissue distribution analysis of NM-104 in rats demonstrated considerable radioactivity present in the thyroid, indicative of _in vivo_ deiodination. Clearly, estrogens would have to be synthesized wherein the radioiodine was incorporated at positions that would not be readily subject to _in vivo_ deiodination.

It was at this stage, that our attention turned to the possible use of nonsteroidal estrogens as the carrier molecules (Fig 3). Diethylstilbestrol (DES) for example, is a potent estrogen and binds very avidly to estrogen receptor protein _in vitro_ (5). Accordingly, iodinated analogs of DES were synthesized, but unfortunately were found to have a low affinity for estrogen receptor protein.

Similar studies were performed in the triphenylethylene series (Fig 4) of which chlorotrianisene is a well-recognized estrogen used clinically. In this series also the tissue distribution results have not been too rewarding (Fig 5). The reasons for this lack of success to date we believe are threefold:

1. The radioiodinated compounds have not exhibited the desired _in vivo_ stability.
2. The analogs do not have sufficient inherent estrogenicity.
3. The radioiodinated compounds have not been of sufficiently high specific activity.

Work is now in progress in an attempt to remedy these deficiencies.

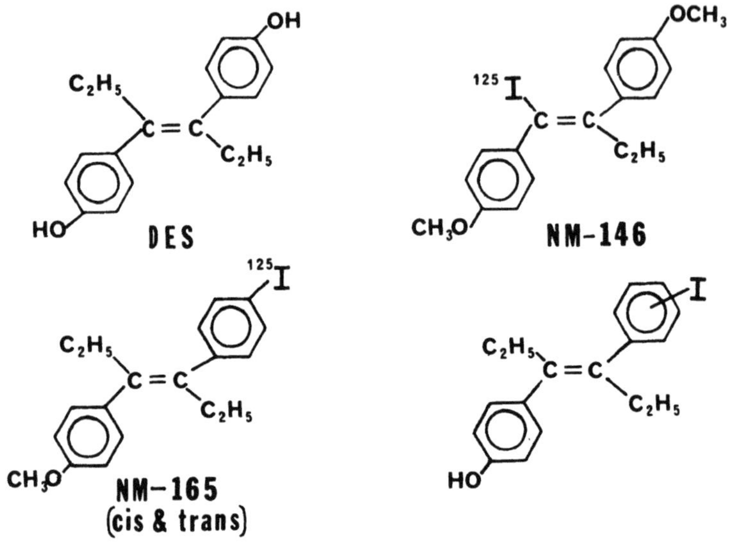

Fig 3. Nonsteroidal Estrogens (Diphenylethylene Series).

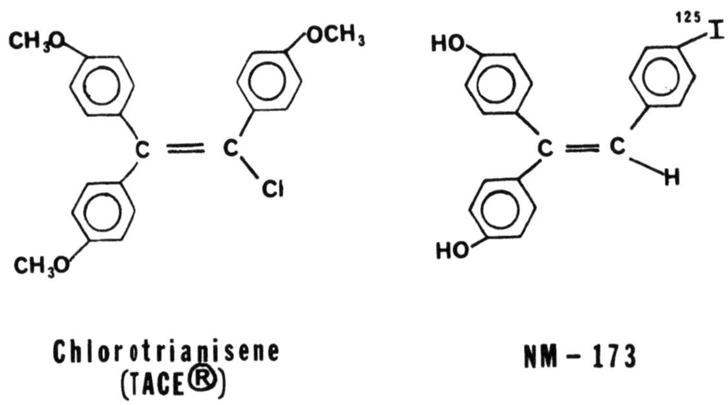

Fig 4. Nonsteroidal Estrogens (Triphenylethylene Series).

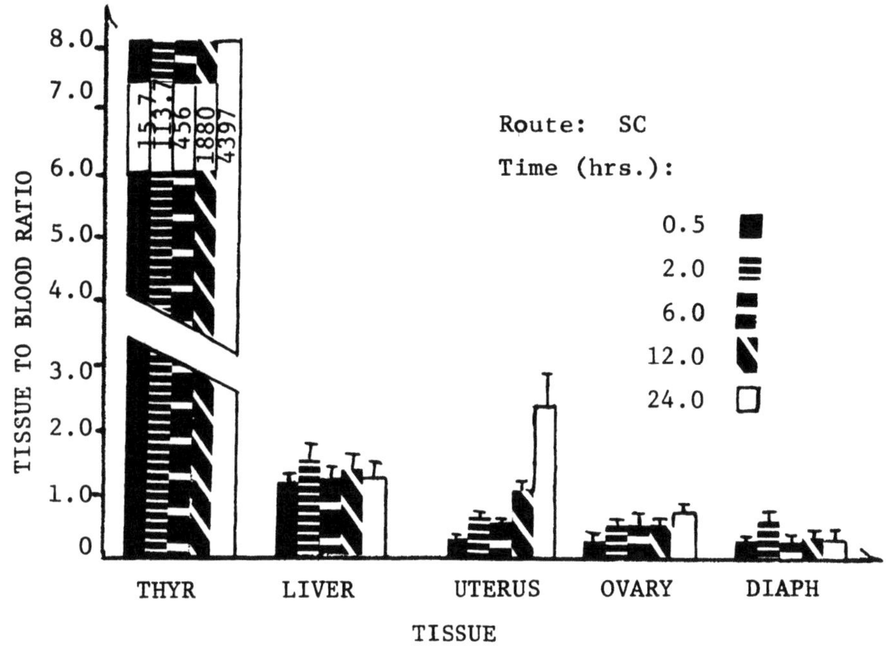

Fig 5. Target to Blood Ratios for Estrogen NM-173 (Sp. Act.= 76 mCi/mg) in Immature Sprague-Dawley Female Rats (± S.E.M.).

As a companion study, we have also been investigating the potential of a radioiodinated antiestrogen as an imaging agent. Antiestrogens have been shown to compete for estrogen binding sites in the target tissues (6) and Schulz and coworkers have shown that the known antiestrogen, clomiphene citrate, selectively accumulates in estrogen responsive tissues in the new born guinea pig. The pituitary levels declined rapidly, but the uterus and liver levels persisted.

We have synthesized several iodinated clomiphene analogs and in one case (NM-177) iodine-125 has been incorporated by isotope exchange (Fig 6). A tritium labelled analog (NM-188) was also prepared by tritiolysis of the aromatically bound iodine. Tissue distribution of these labelled compounds (Fig 7) gave a profile of uptake similar to that previously described for clomiphene citrate. Aside from the thyroid and liver, highest uptake of radioactivity was observed in ovary, pituitary and uterus. Unlike the clomiphene study, however, radioactivity persisted in the ovary and pituitary. There was no major difference in the tissue distribution for the radioiodinated and tritiated analogs.

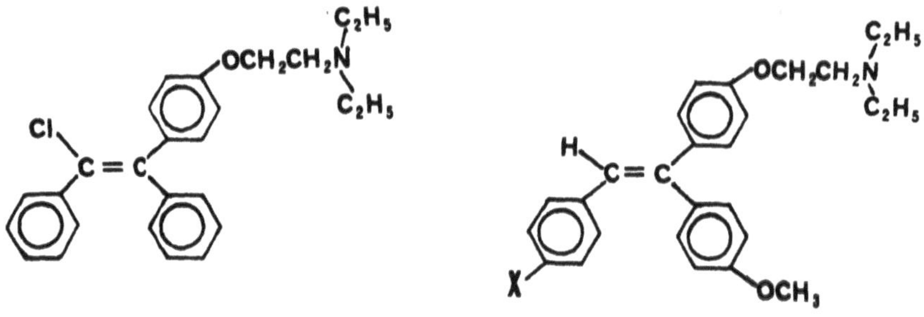

Fig 6. Antiestrogens.

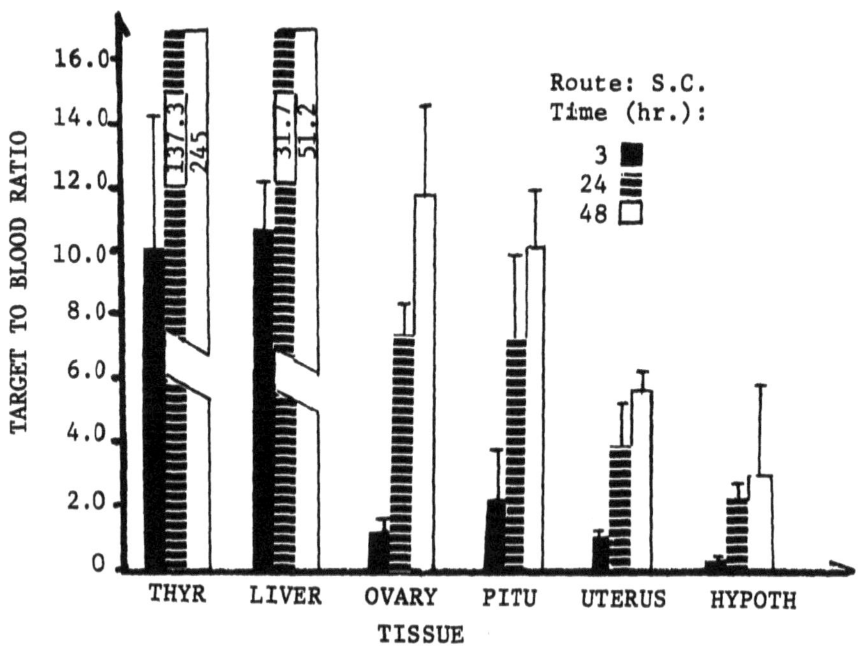

Fig 7. Target to Blood Ratios for Antiestrogen NM-177 (Sp. Act. = 1.2 mCi/mg) in Immature Sprague-Dawley Female Rats (± S.E.M.).

In summary, we look upon these preliminary investigations as discouraging but not disheartening. Obviously the desired agent has not been found, but we certainly believe we are gradually closing in on our goal.

ACKNOWLEDGMENTS

The authors are grateful to Searle Laboratories, Skokie, Illinois for performing the mouse estrogenic assays on compounds prepared in this study and to Professor Lars Terenius, University of Uppsala, Uppsala, Sweden for performing the estrogen receptor protein binding experiments. This work was supported by grant CA-08349 from the National Cancer Institute and funds provided by Searle Laboratories, Skokie, Illinois.

REFERENCES

1. Jensen, E.V. and H.I. Jacobson, Recent Progr. Hormone Res. 18:385, 1962.

2. McGuire, J.L. and R.D. Lisk, Proc. Natl. Acad. Sci., U.S.A. 61:497, 1968.

3. Surks, M.I. and H.C. Shapiro, J. Clin. Endocrinol. Metab. 29:1263, 1969.

4. Mueller, G.P. and W.F. Johns, J. Org. Chem. 26:2403, 1961.

5. Gorski, J., D. Toft, G. Shyamala, D. Smith and A. Notides, Recent Progr. Hormone Res. 24:45, 1968.

6. Wyss, R.H., R. Karsznia, W.L. Heinrichs and W.L. Herrmann, J. Clin. Endocrinol. Metab. 28:1824, 1968.

7. Schulz, K.D., F. Holzel and G. Bettendorf, Acta Endocr. (Kbh) 68:605, 1971.

THE CELLULAR ACTIONS OF GLUCOCORTICOIDS IN RELATION TO HUMAN NEOPLASMS

E. Brad Thompson

Laboratory of Biochemistry, National Cancer Institute
National Institutes of Health
Bethesda, Maryland

Two fundamental concepts concerning the actions of steroid hormones seem to be generally agreed upon. The first is that steroids are inducers, inducers of various specific macromolecules in appropriate target cells. To cite but a few examples, in liver and in certain cultured hepatoma cells, glucocorticoids induce increased synthesis of specific enzymes, such as tryptophan oxygenase and tyrosine aminotransferase (1-3). In immature chicks, estrogens provoke growth, as well as increased specific RNA and protein synthesis (ovalbumin) in target cells (4,5). In rat uterus overall increased growth and specific protein synthesis are induced by estrogen (4,5). Dihydrotestosterone induces several enzymes in rat kidney (6), and progesterone induces avidin in estrogen-primed chick oviduct (7). The list is long (8), and the point seems clear. Steroids are inducers of proteins, DNA, and all the various major classes of RNA. Not all effects are seen in all tissues, of course. The differentiated nature of various cell types defines whether they respond at all to steroids, and if so, to which steroids with which responses. The elements responsible for such specificity and differentiation raise the second fundamental concept in steroid hormone action.

The second concept is that of receptors for steroids. Beginning with studies on estrogen-responsive tissues (9) and by now extended to tissues affected by each class of steroids (10), evidence has been accumulated to show that without exception cells responsive to a particular class of steroid hormone contain receptors specific for that class. These receptors have been found to be proteins with the properties of high affinity, limited capacity, and great specificity for the appropriate type of steroid. In some cases, they have been partially or entirely purified (11-14). They are not found on outer cell membranes, but instead appear to be cytoplasmic, since they remain in the soluble fraction of cell homogenates after high speed centrifugation. They all require protection of thiol groups against oxidation to retain their steroid binding capacity and are further stabilized when steroids are bound to them. These receptor proteins are present in cells which do respond to a steroid hormone, and are absent or present in very low levels in cells which do not respond. Their presence, however, is not always a guarantee of steroid responsiveness (vide intra). After the steroid enters the cell, a process which does not seem to require active transport, it binds to the cytoplasmic receptor, and subsequently undergoes a temperature-dependent alteration to what is often called an activated form. The steps involved in achieving the final active steroid-receptor complex may be multiple and are still the subject of active research (15-17). Nevertheless, at temperatures greater than about 20C, the complex is altered, by processes unknown, to a form that is capable of entering the nucleus and binding to chromatin (9,10). After this has occurred, the specific induced products which the cell is capable of producing begin to appear. The exact means by which the steroid receptor complex evokes these responses still is not known, but in some cases an increased accumulation of functional mRNA for the specific induced protein has been demonstrated. Examples of this include the mRNA's for chick oviduct avidin (18), chick oviduct ovalbumin (18), rat hepatic tryptophan oxygenase (19), and chick retina glutamine synthetase (20), after administration of progesterone, estrogen and dexamethasone, in the appropriate tissue.

At seeming variance with this model of induced cell responses are the known inhibitory effects of glucocorticoids in certain tissues. For many years it has been known that this type of steroid, in supraphysiologic doses at least, suppresses such events as immunoresponsiveness and wound healing. The lympholytic effects of glucocorticoids in particular have been the subject of investigation for decades (21). In rodent thymocytes, glucocorticoids even at quite low concentrations cause inhibition of glucose uptake, of RNA and of DNA synthesis (21). In the embryonic mouse fibroblast line known as L cells (22), similar inhibitory responses have been observed (23). DNA synthesis in rat liver and in some cultured hepatoma cells is inhibited by steroid with corticoid action (24,25), and certain mouse lymphoid cell lines in culture are lysed by glucocorticoids (26). In each of these cases, the responsive cells have been shown to possess receptors specific for active glucocorticoids (27-30), and in the case of L cells and of the cultured mouse lymphoid cells, sub-lines have been isolated which are resistant to these inhibitory effects. In many cases, these resistant lines have been shown to have lost all or much of their receptor content, or to have receptors with lowered affinity for glucocorticoids (26,30-36). In fact, these findings have bolstered the view that the receptor proteins are indeed an obligatory first step in steroid action.

The seeming paradox, that steroids are inducing agents in some cells, inhibitory compounds in others, and both inhibitors and inducers in yet others, in each case acting through receptors with apparently the same properties, has not been definitively resolved. Some evidence, however, suggests that even the inhibitory effects are secondary to inductive processes. Thus, for example, in rat thymocytes the steroid-evoked reduction in thymidine incorporation and other cellular processes can be blocked by inhibitors of macromolecular synthesis (37-40). Consequently, the model has been proposed that steroids may be inducing some molecule or process which proves inhibitory or even lethal to the cell.

GLUCOCORTICOID EFFECTS IN LEUKEMIC LYMPHOBLASTS

The data that receptors represented a necessary early step in the inhibitory effects of glucocorticoids in appropriate lines of tissue culture cells led us to the idea of examining appropriate types of cells from human diseases for receptors. Early studies by Jensen and his collaborators had given encouragement to the view that quantification of estrogen receptors in tumor cells from breast cancer patients would prove of predictive value for the effectiveness of therapeutic endocrine manipulations (41), studies which subsequently have been amply confirmed (42). We decided to examine, therefore, cells from patients with leukemia. Glucocorticoids have long been known to be of value in the treatment of certain leukemias, but in the days of single drug therapy, the remissions they induced were not complete or permanent, and indeed in some types of leukemia, such as acute myelogenous leukemia (AML), improvement was observed only in sporadic cases (43-46). Various tests had been applied to leukemic cells, attempting to predict their usefulness in specific cases, but these had proved of only limited value for various reasons (47-50). Treatment with high-dose corticosteroids may result in many undesirable side effects, including Cushing's syndrome, gastric ulcer, suppression of immune responsiveness, heightened risk of infection, psychosis, etc. Since these profound effects of the high dosage courses of steroids often included in modern therapy of the leukemias would be best avoided, it seemed of value to examine cells from leukemic patients for glucocorticoid receptors to see whether their presence would correlate with a favorable response. Besides, at that time no experiments had shown a functional role for glucocorticoid receptors in human cells, and thus the opportunity for establishing such a link presented itself. The technique of leukophoresis, applied in the treatment of many patients in the leukemia service at the National Institutes of Health, along with the storage of viable cells by freezing in dimethyl sulfoxide, provided us with quantities of leukemic cells sufficient to carry out the studies. First it was necessary to establish the validity of the assay system and to determine whether, in fact, corticosteroid receptors could be demonstrated in human leukemic blasts. Preliminary studies on selected lines of rodent leukemic cells and on fresh rodent thymocytes indicated that the assay methods employed could detect receptors in cells known to contain them. In the human cell the main receptor assay used, one based on the ability of non-radioactive steroid to compete for binding at the specific receptor sites, was verified.

The competitive binding assay used in these experiments depends on the comparison of paired cell extracts, both of which are incubated with a given concentration of radioactive steroid (Fig 1). To one member of the pair, a large excess of non-radioactive steroid is added as well. The assay depends on the fact that in most

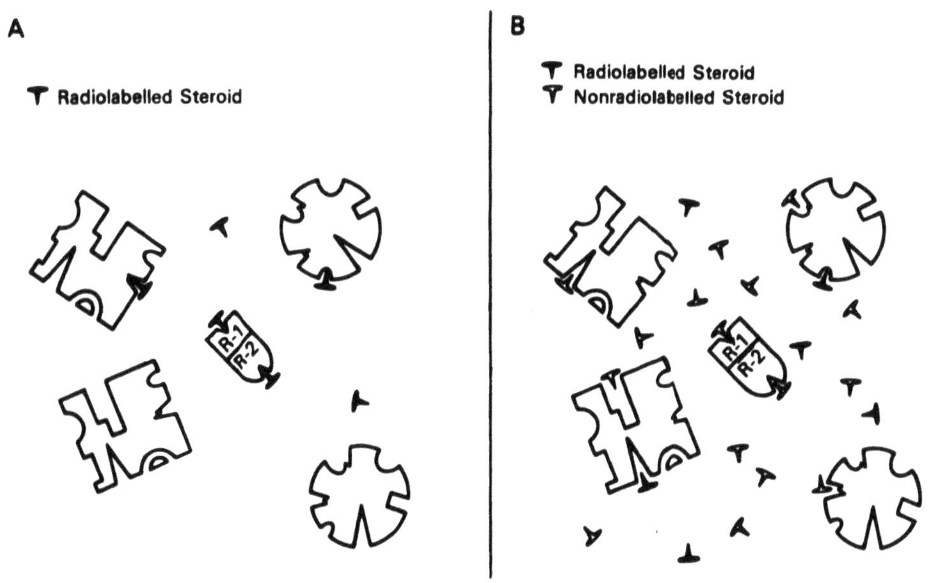

Fig 1. Model for competitive binding assay used in estimating steroid receptor content of cells. Receptor molecule with two binding sites R-1 and R-2 shown in center. Non-specific binding sites shown surrounding.

crude cell extracts, a very large number of proteins bind steroids weakly and non-specifically. Thus adding more steroid competes only with the radiolabelled hormone at the specific receptor sites, since they are limited in number. The non-specific sites, however, bind both radiolabelled and unlabelled steroid equally well; these sites are "not competible". In order for the assay accurately to reflect specific sites, therefore, it is necessary to show empirically in a newly examined system that the above facts hold true. This was done for the leukemic lymphoblasts, and linearity of response for specific binding sites over the range of extract protein concentrations used was demonstrated as well (51).

With these essential preliminaries complete, we examined the nature of the receptors in the blasts from a series of patients with acute lymphoblastic leukemia, ALL (51,52). Diagnosis had been established at NIH by standard criteria. The cells for these studies were from patients under 30 years of age who had received no glucocorticoid therapy within 10 days of cell collection. Radiolabelled cortisol or the synthetic glucocorticoid dexamethasone was used in these studies, usually the latter because of its very low affinity for human corticosteroid binding globulin (CBG). This choice therefore ensures against including contaminating serum CBG in measurements of cellular steroid receptors. Fig 2 shows the results of a study on extracts of one patient's cells. The data shown demonstrate both total and specific (competible) binding. The inset depicts the data in the form of a Scatchard plot, from which an apparent dissociation constant (-1/slope) and number of sites (x-intercept) can be derived (53). Thus in the cell extract shown, about 0.2 pmol/mg protein of specific, saturable sites were found, the apparent dissociation constant was 0.3×10^{-8}M and the number of binding sites per cell was about 1.5×10^{3}. The single straight line fitting the data points indicated a single class of sites. The apparent dissociation constant using dexamethasone as the test steroid was calculated to be 7×10^{-9}M. Both in quantity and affinity, these values were similar to those which had been found in other, non-human cells. These assays, of course, were carried out at 0-4° because the receptor's binding capability is rapidly lost at 37°. The affinities of intracellular receptors at body temperature therefore cannot be directly obtained by these methods. Nevertheless they do give a useful indication of the affinity of receptor for steroid.

Kinetic studies were next carried out on cell extracts from a patient for whom sufficient cells were available. Rates of association and dissociation of steroid with specific sites were determined. The data obtained were consistent with second order kinetics for the binding reaction:

$$\text{steroid} + \text{receptor} \longrightarrow (\text{steroid-receptor complex}),$$

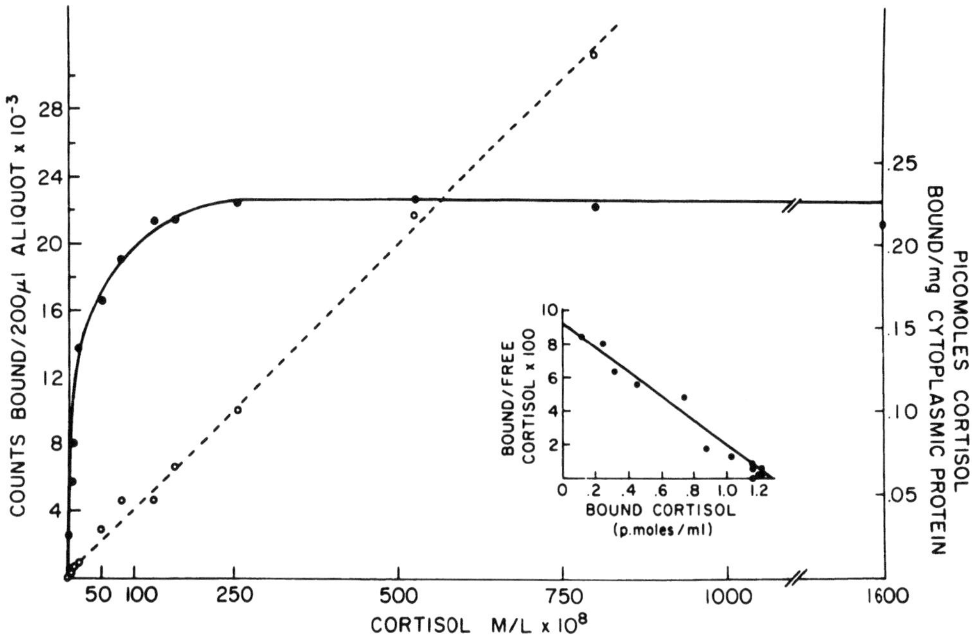

Fig 2. Binding of ^{3}H cortisol in an extract from human ALL lymphoblasts. Closed circles, specific binding. Open circles, nonspecific binding. Insert, Scatchard plot of specific binding. From Ref. 51.

and first order kinetics for the dissociation

$$\text{(complex)} \longrightarrow \text{receptor} + \text{steroid.}$$

The overall equilibrium constant calculated from these experiments was 0.5×10^{-9}M for dexamethasone, in reasonable agreement with the value of 7×10^{-9}M obtained from the competitive binding Scatchard technique. Thus it seemed that these cells could contain steroid receptors with qualities similar to those described for animal cells. The next experiments were designed to test the receptor for steroid specificity and cellular specificity.

Steroid specificity was examined by testing the ability of a variety of steroids to compete with radiolabelled dexamethasone in the binding assay. In these experiments, ^{3}H dexamethasone, 3.8×10^{-7}M, was added to each of a series of aliquots of lymphoblast extract, and non-radioactive steroids (each at 3.8×10^{-5}M) were added to different samples (Table I). The ability of each steroid to compete for specific binding sites was compared to that of non-radiolabelled dexamethasone itself. As the table shows, active glucocorticoids compete well, less active ones less well, and non-glucocorticoids not at all. Some compounds, such as progesterone and cortexolone, shown to be antagonistic to glucocorticoids in lymphoid cell systems (5,4), compete relatively well.

Cell specificity was examined using tests aimed at correlating receptor site saturation with cellular responses to corticoids. Cells were exposed to various concentrations of glucocorticoid for 18 hours at 37° in tissue culture medium, followed by a two hour exposure to radiolabelled thymidine or uridine. Extracts of the

TABLE I

Specificity of Glucocorticoid Receptor Activity in Leukemic Cell Extracts

Competing Steroid (100 fold excess)	(% Inhibition of ^{3}H Dexamethasone Binding) ALL*	AML*
Dexamethasone	Set at 100	Set at 100
Hydrocortisone	100	98
Prednisolone	78	100
Aldosterone	88	95
Triamcinolone	94	95
Progesterone	100	ND†
5β-dihydrocortisol	100	ND†
Deoxycorticosterone	76	72
Corticosterone	76	65
Cortexolone	69	ND†
2α-hydroxycortisol	60	ND†
17α-methyl testosterone	60	28
Spironolactone	43	ND†
Prednisone	31	48
Testosterone	26	ND†
19-Nortestosterone	16	54
Cortisone	16	ND†
17α-Estradiol	6	39
Etiocholanolone	0	13
Tetrahydrocortisol	0	3
Androstenedione	0	ND†

*Data from References 51 and 57.
ND, test not done.

same cells not previously treated with steroid were assayed for their levels of receptor binding of corticoid across the same range of concentrations. By comparing the two dose-response curves, one could see whether a correlation existed between the concentration of hormone which saturated the receptor (at 4° in a cell-free extract) and that which evoked a cell response (at 37°). Table 2 left hand side, shows the results of such an experiment. Considering the differing assay conditions, there does seem to be a good correlation, with maximum binding in this extract and maximum inhibition of thymidine uptake both occurring around 2-4 x 10^{-7}M dexamethasone. Thymidine incorporation was inhibited in all five of the untreated patients studied who had steroid receptors. In contrast, a few patients' cells had much less or no receptor by the competitive binding assay. In these patients, where quantities of cells permitted, we also tested for inhibition of thymidine uptake after exposure to corticosteroids. Table 2, right hand side, shows the results of such an experiment. First, note that there was very little in the way of active receptor molecules in the extract. The levels of specific binding were about 10% of those seen in the extract from the sensitive cells. (They can be compared directly, even though the data are expressed as cpm/aliquot, because the protein content of the extracts was nearly identical.) Furthermore, as is immediately apparent, there was no inhibition of thymidine uptake across the concentration range tested.

From these experiments, we conclude that specific glucocorticoid receptors exist in the lymphoblasts of some patients with acute lymphoblastic leukemia and not in others. These receptors seem to be necessary for active steroids to exert their inhibitory effects on the cells <u>in vitro</u>. At present, we cannot tell whether the low levels of binding in the resistant cells are due to a small subpopulation of cells with a complete complement of receptors, to a lowered receptor content in all cells, to an altered receptor with lower steroid affinity, or whether each of these mechanisms may be found in different patients.

Clinical correlations, done in retrospect, suggest that measurement of glucocorticoid receptors may be useful in predicting therapeutic response. Twenty-two previously treated patients with ALL were all found to have significant levels of glucocorticoid receptors in their lymphoblasts, viz., 0.1-0.6 pmol/mg protein. All these patients responded to combination therapy which included high dose corticosteroids (Table 3). Six patients in relapse who subsequently responded to the same therapy also had cells with receptor levels in the same range. Six other patients in relapse who had had little or no measurable receptor were those who failed to respond to therapy. As the table shows, normal peripheral lymphocytes also had virtually no receptor, data which fits with other reports of their lack of sensitivity to steroids in <u>in vitro</u> tests (47,55),

Table 2

Comparison *In Vitro* of Cytosol Steroid Receptor Binding with Inhibition of Thymidine Uptake in ALL Lymphoblasts as a Function of Dexamethasone Concentration

	Patient Clinically Responsive[2]		Patient Clinically Resistant[2]	
[^{3}H Dexamethasone]	cpm steroid bound per 200μl cytosol[3]	% Inhibition ^{3}H Thymidine Uptake[4]	cpm steroid bound per 200μl cytosol	% Inhibition
0	----	0%	----	0%
5×10^{-8}M	2000cpm	30	120cpm	0
1×10^{-7}	3100	55	150	0
2×10^{-7}	3700	65	250	0
4×10^{-7}	4000	70	375	0
7×10^{-7}	4000	70	375	0
2.6×10^{-6}	3700	70	----	---

1) All data calculated from Reference 51.

2) Clinically responsive patient had had no prior treatment. Remission was produced by combined therapy, including glucocorticoids. Virtually identical results were obtained in cells from a total of 5 such patients. Clinically resistant patient had obtained one or more remissions after prior treatment but at this relapse failed to respond. Four such patients gave similar results. No patient had received glucocorticoids for at least 10 days before study.

3) These are "competible counts" in standard charcoal assays.

4) Thymidine uptake after 2 hr exposure as trichloroacetic acid precipitable material.

TABLE 3

Steroid Receptor Levels in the Cytoplasm of Lymphoblasts from Patients with Acute Lymphoblastic Leukemia*

Clinical Status (No. of Individuals)	Receptor pmol dexamethasone specifically bound per mg protein ± SD
Untreated (22)	0.31 ± 0.1
Previously treated, still sensitive to combined therapy including steroids (6)	0.30 ± 0.12
Previously treated, now resistant (6)	0.015 ± 0.0095

*Derived from data in Reference 51.

and may help to explain their insensitivity to therapeutic doses of corticoids *in vivo*.

Acute myelogenous leukemia (AML) is a disease with a quite different history of clinical response to steroid therapy. Frequently, there is little or no response; yet a few patients appear to improve (43,56). Accordingly, we examined cells of sixteen patients with this form of leukemia for the presence of receptor as well as typical *in vitro* responses (57). Three of the sixteen patients' cells were found to contain receptors by the competitive assay. One of the three appeared similar to what had been seen in all the ALL cells, with specific binding in the extract showing saturation at about 2 x 10^{-7}M dexamethasone. In thymidine uptake experiments, this patient's cells showed maximum inhibition of uptake at a similar concentration (Fig 3). Steroid specificity studies as in the ALL cases showed that this binding was restricted to steroids with glucocorticoid or anti-glucocorticoid activity (Table 1). The two other patients whose cell extracts contained corticosteroid binding activity required much higher steroid concentrations to achieve saturation, approximately 10^{-6}M.

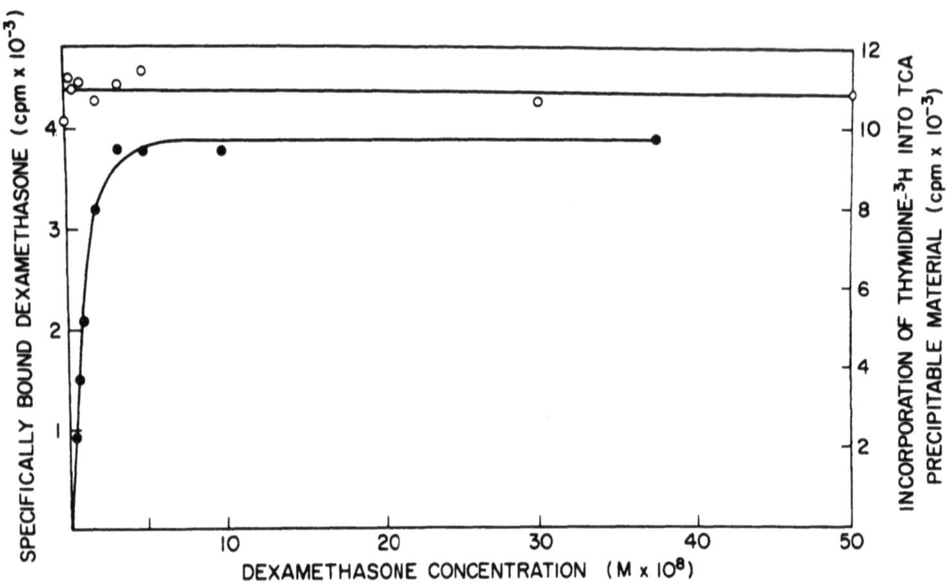

Fig 3. Specific binding of dexamethasone in cytoplasmic extracts from the blasts of a patient with AML (closed circles), compared with ^3H thymidine incorporation in whole cells into trichloroacetic acid precipitable material (open circles). Both variables shown as a function of dexamethasone concentration. From Reference 57.

The remaining thirteen AML patients showed little or no corticosteroid binding activity in extracts from their blasts. As with some of the ALL patients, some of the AML patients showed a little binding activity, perhaps 1/10 - 1/15 of the levels seen in of Fig 3. The same speculations as for the ALL cases concerning the origin of this residual activity apply. Cells of the AML patients with little or no receptor were tested for their _in vitro_ responses to glucocorticoids. No effect was found in six cases tested for inhibition of uridine and/or thymidine uptake and four cases tested for inhibition of glucose utilization (58). Clinical data was not available for the AML patients. Similar data had been obtained in six AML patients' cells by Gailani et al, who found in only two of the six cases studied evidence for specific glucocorticoid binding. The same group found receptors in 3 of 3 ALL cases examined and in

4 of 4 lymphosarcomas, but none in any of 8 chronic lymphocytic and 2 of chronic myelocytic leukemic cells (59).

The aim of these studies was to see whether knowing the quantity of glucocorticoid receptors in human leukemic blasts might be of use in predicting the response of patients to such hormones. Our results give encouragement to this view.

Although the data in these studies on cells obtained directly from patients is encouraging, more data, including prospective studies should be obtained before a final conclusion can be made. Various tests have been applied to leukemic cells to assess steroid effects and predict therapeutic response (47-50). None have proven to be uniformly successful. It is not clear that any single test will be sufficient to predict such a response with complete accuracy. Cline has used methods such as thymidine uptake to test steroid toxicity for leukemic cells (48,49). Functional tests such as this should be excellent; however, Cline's experiments were carried out with quite high steroid concentrations and thus may have shown effects due to steroid levels well above those which can be achieved therapeutically. It is noteworthy in the cells we have studied that the receptors are saturated, and thymidine incorporation inhibited, at around 2×10^{-7}M dexamethasone or even higher concentrations of cortisol. This would explain why the circulating corticosteroids in these leukemic patients do not effect a self-cure. It is now generally agreed that it is the free and not the total (including protein-bound) steroid which is the effective substance (60). Recent estimates of free circulating cortisol place its diurnal range between about 7.6×10^{-9}M and 5×10^{-8}M. ACTH could evoke levels of about 1.5×10^{-7}M (61). Thus only by therapeutic administration of potent and long-acting corticosteroids can one expect to saturate the receptors in the leukemic cells for a long enough period to produce inhibitory effects. The most reliable indicator of therapeutic response may be a combined examination of receptor content and some functional response at appropriate steroid concentrations.

Measuring receptor content alone may not be sufficient. In the many studies on breast cancer patients, lack of estrogen receptors shows a high correlation with lack of response, but the presence of estrogen receptors only predicts success of appropriate endocrine therapy in about 60% of the patients (42). Several reasons may account for this. First, it is possible in a disease such as breast cancer, that the receptor content of the tissue examined may differ from that in metastases elsewhere in the body, although direct data from assays on multiple site biopsies suggest that this is not the usual explanation (42). Second, it may be that the tumor consists of a mixture of cells, some steroid-sensitive and receptor-containing, and others without receptors and therefore steroid-insensitive. Assays on such a mixture would of course indicate the presence of receptors. Third, some cells may contain measurable receptors which nevertheless do not function properly. Fourth, tumor cells might contain normal receptors but be blocked in their steroid-receptor binding and movement into the nucleus. Finally, all the above may be normal but the cell responses blocked at an even later step. We have recently obtained evidence for this latter class in a line of glucocorticoid - not estrogen - responsive cells, HTC cells. In certain subclones of these cells, the enzyme tyrosine aminotransferase, normally inducible by physiologic concentrations of glucocorticoids, no longer can be induced. Basal levels of the enzyme are still present, and by any of the several parameters tested so far, cellular glucocorticoid receptors are normal (Thompson, Aviv and Lippman, manuscript submitted for publication).

In the case of the human leukemias, we have not as yet found an acute lymphoblastic leukemia patient with cellular receptors who failed to respond to therapy which included steroids (see above). However, the possibility of finding receptor-positive cells from a patient with one or another form of steroid resistant leukemia certainly exists. The first possiblity mentioned above in the context of breast cancer, mixed metastases, seems unlikely. However, any of the other four are possible. Kaiser et al have reported that resistant lines of the transplantable mouse lymphosarcoma P1798 show somewhat reduced amounts of receptor with normal steroid affinity (62). They postulate that the resistant tumors are composed of a mixture of receptor-containing sensitive cells and receptor-lacking insensitive cells. In cultured lines of mouse lymphoid cells, steroid-resistant clones have been found which contain easily detectable but subtly altered receptors (33,34,63).

In the case of human cells, we have reported on two cell lines in long-term culture which contained apparently normal cytoplasmic receptors but which were found to be insensitive to killing by steroids (64). These cells contained specific glucocorticoid receptors as judged by competition studies similar to those described above. The concentration of cytoplasmic receptors in cell homogenates was 0.7 and 0.9 pmol dexamethasone bound per mg cell protein, at or above the high end of the usual range, and the affinity seemed similar to that for other leukemic blasts. When steroid-charged, heat-activated extracts from these cells were incubated with nuclei, transfer of radioactivity into the nuclear fraction occurred as expected for a steroid-responsive system (Fig 4). However these same cells, when examined for typical inhibitory responses to steroids, were found to be resistant. Fig 5 shows the saturation curve for dexamethasone binding, compared with the thymidine uptake into acid precipitable material. As can readily be seen, there is no inhibition of thymidine uptake despite a normal-appearing receptor curve. Similar lack of response was found for uridine uptake and glucose utilization. Of course, these cells had been grown in culture for

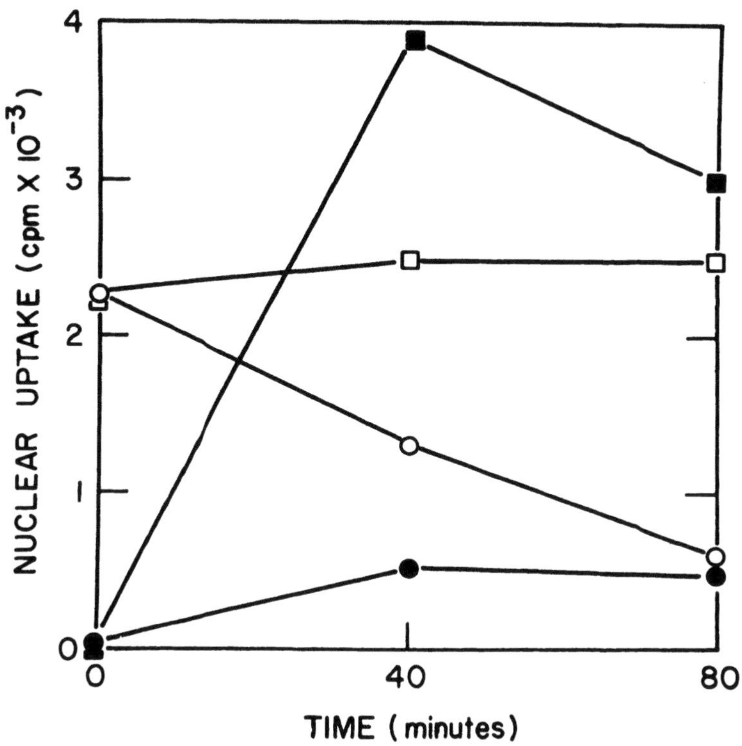

Fig 4. Nuclear binding of cytoplasmic steroid-receptor complexes. Cytosol and nuclei were preincubated at 0° in buffer containing ^3H dexamethasone with or without 100-fold excess of nonradioactive dexamethasone. At time 0, nuclei and cytosols were mixed. Those preincubated with ^3H dexamethasone only were combined, and those preincubated with radioactive dexamethasone plus excess nonradioactive dexamethasone were combined. Each combination was divided and incubated at 0° or 20°, samples being taken at various times. Specifically bound radioactivity, determined by difference is plotted. Nuclei at 0° shown by closed circles and nuclei at 20° shown by open squares and cytosol at 20° by open circles. As can be seen at 20° but not at 0° there is a loss of radioactivity from the cytosol and uptake by the nuclei. From Reference 64.

some time, and perhaps the culture conditions had resulted in the development of steroid resistance. Nevertheless, these results lead us to predict that as more cases of leukemia are examined, some will be found which possess receptors but nevertheless are steroid resistant. Our experience to date with cells fresh from patients suggests that such cases will be the exception.

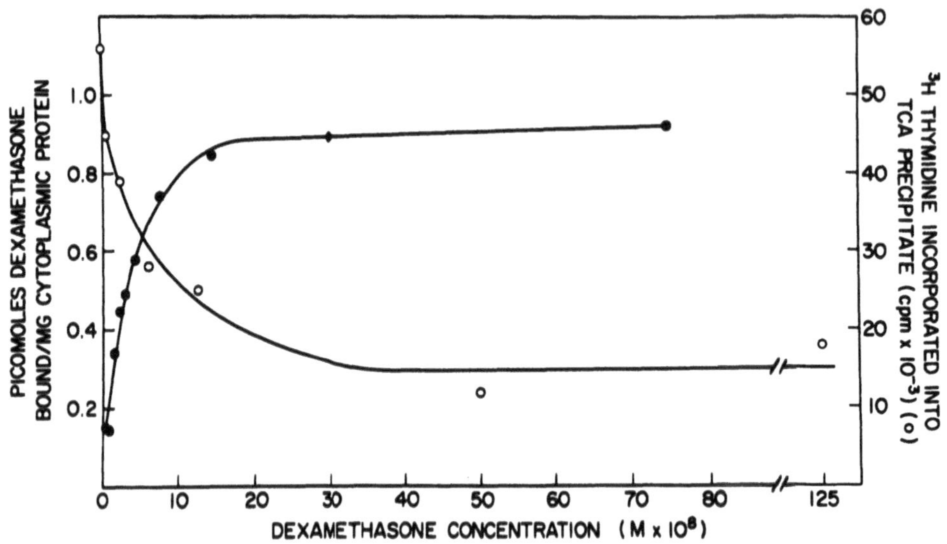

Fig 5. Comparison of ^{3}H dexamethasone binding and ^{3}H thymidine uptake, as in Fig 3. In this case cells were a cultured line derived from a patient with ALL. From Reference 64.

In sum, measurement of steroid receptors in the leukemias holds promise as a means of predicting <u>in vivo</u> response to hormonal therapy. Perhaps the best test would be one combining some measure of receptor content with a measure of functional response, done at levels of free steroid expected in therapy. In addition, studies of steroid receptors seem to be providing a clue to the mechanism by which most leukemias escape from steroid responsiveness. This most commonly appears to be by developing a population of cells which lack receptors. Whether this end result is due to selection of a receptorless cell population which already exists in the patient, or whether the steroid or other drugs generate such a population remains to be seen.

REFERENCES

1. Lin, E.C.C. and W.E. Knox, Biochim. Biophys. Acta 26:85, 1957.

2. Kenney, F.T., J. Biol. Chem. 237:1610, 1962.

3. Thompson, E.B., G.M. Tomkins and J.F. Curran, Proc. Natl. Acad. Sci., U.S.A. 56:296, 1966.

4. O'Malley, B.W., New Engl. J. Med. 284:370, 1971.

5. Palmiter, R.D., T. Oka and R.T. Schimke, J. Biol. Chem. 246:724, 1971.

6. Paigen, K., R.T. Swank, S. Tomino and R.E. Ganschow, J. Cell Physiol. 85:379, 1975.

7. Korenman, S.G. and B.W. O'Malley, Endocrinology 83:11, 1968.

8. Pitot, H.C. and M.B. Yatvin, Physiol. Rev. 53:228, 1973.

9. Jensen, E.V., S. Mohla, T.A. Gorell and E.R. DeSombre, Vitamins and Hormones 32:89, 1974.

10. King, R.J.B. and W.I.P. Mainwaring, Steroid-Cell Interactions, Univ. Park Press, Baltimore, 1974, p. 430.

11. DeSombre, E.R., J.P. Chaband, G.A. Puca and E.V. Jensen, J. Steroid Biochem. 3:445, 1972.

12. Jensen, E.V., S. Mohla, T. Gorell, S. Tanaka and E.R. De Sombre, J. Steroid Biochem. 3:445, 1972.

13. Failla, D., G.M. Tomkins and D.V. Santi, Proc. Natl. Acad. Sci., U.S.A. 72:3849, 1975.

14. Schrader, W.T. and B.W. O'Malley, J. Biol. Chem. 247:51, 1972.

15. Rousseau, G.G., J.D. Baxter and G.M. Tomkins, J. Mol. Biol. 67:99, 1972.

16. Pratt, W.B., J.L. Kaine and D.V. Pratt, J. Biol. Chem. 250: 4584, 1975.

17. Mosher, K.M., D.A. Young and A. Munck, J. Biol. Chem. 246: 654, 1971.

18. Chan, L., A.R. Means and B.W. O'Malley, Proc. Natl. Acad. Sci., U.S.A. 70:1870, 1973.

19. Schutz, G., G. Killewich, G. Chen and P. Feigelson, Proc. Natl. Acad. Sci., U.S.A. 72:1017, 1975.

20. Schwartz, R.J., Nature New Biol. 237:121, 1972.

21. Makman, M.H., S. Nakagawa and A. White, Rec. Progr. Horm. Res. 23:195, 1967.

22. Earle, W.R., J. Nat. Cancer Inst. 4:165, 1943.

23. Pratt, W.B. and L. Aronow, J. Biol. Chem. 241:5244, 1966.

24. Henderson, I.C., R.E. Fischel and J.N. Loeb, Endocrinology 88:1471, 1971.

25. Loeb, J.N., C. Borek and L.L. Yeung, Proc. Natl. Acad. Sci., U.S.A. 70:3852, 1973.

26. Rosenau, W., J.D. Baxter, G.G. Rousseau and G.M. Tomkins, Nature New Biol. 237:20, 1972.

27. Kirkpatrick, A.F., R.J. Milholland and F. Rosen, Nature New Biol. 232:216, 1971.

28. Munck, A.C. Wira, D.A. Young, K.M. Mosher, C. Hallahan and P.A. Bell, J. Steroid Biochem. 3:567, 1972.

29. Hackney, J.F., S.R. Gross, L. Aronow and W.B. Pratt, Mol. Pharmacol. 6:500, 1970.

30. Baxter, J.D., A.W. Harris, G.M. Tomkins and M. Cohn, Science 171:189, 1971.

31. Aronow, L. and J.D. Gabourel, Proc. Soc. Exp. Biol. Med. 111: 348, 1962.

32. Kirkpatrick, A.F., R.J. Milholland and F. Rosen, Nature New Biol. 232:216, 1971.

33. Kaiser, N., R.J. Milholland and F. Rosen, Cancer Res. 34: 621, 1974.

34. Sibley, C.H. and G.M. Tomkins, Cell 2:213 and 221, 1974.

35. Lippman, M.E. and E.B. Thompson, J. Biol. Chem. 249:2483, 1974.

36. Pratt, W.B. and D.N. Ishii, Biochem. 11:1401, 1972.

37. Mosher, K.M., D.A. Young and A. Munck, J. Biol. Chem. 246: 654, 1971.

38. Makman, M.H., B. Dvorkin and A. White, Proc. Natl. Acad. Sci., U.S.A. 68:1269, 1971.

39. Makman, M.H., B. Dvorkin and A. White, J. Biol. Chem. 245: 2556, 1970.

40. White, A. and M.H. Makman, Adv. Enz. Res. 5:317, 1967.

41. Jensen, E.V., G.E. Block, S. Smith, K. Kyser and E.R. DeSombre, Nat. Cancer Inst. Monograph 34:55, 1971.

42. McGuire, W.L., P.P. Carbone and E.P. Vollmer (eds), Estrogen Receptors in Human Breast Cancer, Raven Press, New York, 1975.

43. Ranney, H. and A. Gellhorn, Amer. J. Med. 22:405, 1957.

44. Granville, N., F. Rubio, Jr., A. Unugur, E. Schulman and W. Dameshek, New Engl. J. Med. 259:207, 1958.

45. Shanbrom, E. and S. Miller, New Engl. J. Med. 266:1354, 1962.

46. Henderson, E.S., Semin. Hematol. 6:271, 1969.

47. Schrek, R., J. Natl. Cancer Inst. 33:837, 1964.

48. Cline, M.J. and E. Rosenbaum, Cancer Res. 28:2516, 1968.

49. Cline, M.J., Blood 30:176, 1967.

50. Werthamer, S. and L. Amaral, Blood 37:463, 1971.

51. Lippman, M.E., R.H. Halterman, B.G. Leventhal, S. Perry and E.B. Thompson, J. Clin. Invest. 52:1715, 1973.

52. Lippman, M.E., R. Halterman, S. Perry, B. Leventhal and E.B. Thompson, Nature New Biol. 242:157, 1973.

53. Scatchard, G., Ann. N.Y. Acad. Sci. 51:660, 1949.

54. Munck, A. and C. Wira, In: Raspe, G. (ed.), Advances in the Biosciences 7, Schering Workshop on Steroid Hormone Receptors, Pergamon Press, New York, 1971, p. 301.

55. Claman, H.N., J.W. Moorhead and W.H. Benner, J. Lab. Clin. Med. 78:499, 1971.

56. Roath, S., M. Israels, J. Wilkinson, Quart. J. Med. 33:257, 1964.

57. Lippman, M.E., S. Perry and E.B. Thompson, Amer. J. Med. 59: 224, 1975.

58. Munck, A., Perspect. Biol. Med. 14:265, 1971.

59. Gailani, S., J. Minowada, P. Silvernail, A. Nussbaum, N. Kaiser, F. Rosen and K. Shimaoka, Cancer Res. 33:2653, 1973.

60. Yates, F.E., D.J. Marsh and J.W. Maran, In: Mountcastle, (ed.), Medical Physiology, Vol. 2, The C.V. Mosby Co., St. Louis, 1974, p. 1696.

61. Baumann, G., G. Rappaport, T. Lemarchand-Berand and J. Felber, J. Clin. Endocrinol. Metab. 40:462, 1975.

62. Kaiser, N., R.J. Milholland and F. Rosen, Cancer Res. 34: 621, 1974.

63. Yamamoto, K.R., M.R. Stampfer and G.M. Tomkins, Proc. Natl. Acad. Sci., U.S.A. 71:3901, 1974.

64. Lippman, M.E., S. Perry and E.B. Thompson, Cancer Res. 34: 1572, 1974.

ADRENAL STEROIDS, MEMBRANES AND NEOPLASIA

Thomas D. Gelehrter

Departments of Human Genetics and Internal Medicine
University of Michigan
Ann Arbor, Michigan

Neoplastic cells show qualitative differences from normal cells in their overall patterns of gene expression (1); in particular, malignant transformation has been shown to involve a number of structural and functional alterations in the cell membrane (2-8). The plasma membrane may play a vital role in the regulation of cell division by affecting the transport of essential nutrients into the cell, and by acting as the transmitter and transducer of signals arising from cell-cell interactions. Uncontrolled growth could result from abnormalities in transport regulation, or in aberrant sensitivity to external signals which normally regulate cell division (2,8).

A variety of differences in membrane structure and function have been described between transformed and normal cells in tissue culture (2-8). These include: a) loss of density-dependent inhibition of growth when cells undergo malignant transformation, resulting in an increased saturation density; b) ability to grow without anchorage dependence reflected as an ability to grow in agar, in suspension culture, or in methylcellulose; c) decreased adhesiveness to a substratum as well as to other cells, a change which may be important in the process of metastasis; d) increased agglutinability by a variety of plant lectins; e) increased rate of transport of sugars and amino acids; f) altered morphology, both in gross shape and in cell surface microarchitecture; g) change in the chemical composition of the membrane, particularly affecting glycoproteins; h) change in the antigenic nature of the cell membrane, resulting in the expression of determinants usually present only in embryonic cells; and i) enhanced production of proteases, such as plasminogen activator. Although these alterations in membrane phenotype have been described in a variety of transformed cells, they are not invariable or necessary markers of the neoplastic state. Furthermore, with the exception of the antigenic changes resulting from the expression of viral antigens in virally-transformed cells, the other changes most probably represent alterations in the expression of cellular genes secondary to neoplastic transformation. Certain normal cells may also demonstrate some of the membrane changes considered typical of neoplastic cells (9), and some of these phenotypic features may be seen in normal cells only during specific phases of the cell cycle (10).

Of particular interest is the finding that environmental agents can also affect the membrane phenotype in a manner similar or opposite to neoplastic transformation. Thus, the addition of serum or insulin to resting normal cells can overcome density-dependent inhibition of growth (2,8). On the other hand, incubation of transformed fibroblastic lines (11) or Chinese hamster ovary cells (12) with cyclic AMP results in a "reverse transformation" in which the cells lose their malignant phenotype and take on a more normal phenotype. For example, the incubation of Chinese hamster ovary cells, a permanent line of epithelioid cells, with 1 mM dibutyryl cyclic AMP results in a rapid alteration of morphology toward that of normal fibroblasts, associated with oriented, monolayer growth exhibiting strict density-dependent inhibition (although growth rate and cloning efficiency are not significantly changed). In addition, the cells show changes in surface morphology, changes in membrane glycoproteins, and a decreased ability to be agglutinated by plant lectins. Testosterone propionate potentiates the effect of dibutyryl cyclic AMP as do prostaglandins, but estrogens, glucocorticoids, epinephrine, glucagon, and insulin are without effect. The mechanism of this reverse transformation is unknown, but appears to involve microtubules and microfilament structures in that it is inhibited by colcemid and cytochalasin B (12,13).

Recently, our laboratory has obtained evidence that adrenal steroids can also bring about a program similar to reverse transformation in a permanent line of rat hepatoma cells (HTC) in tissue culture. These studies were initiated because of our interest in the induction of the enzyme tyrosine aminotransferase by glucocorticoids and insulin (14,15). We decided to assess the role of amino acid transport in the hormonal effects on specific protein synthesis by studying the transport of the non-metabolized amino acid analogue, α-aminoisobutyric acid (AIB). AIB is transported in a number of tissues by the so-called A or alanine-preferring system for neutral amino acids (16). HTC cells actively transport AIB against a concentration gradient by a saturable, energy-dependent process. A single transport system which exhibits Michaelis-Menten kinetics appears to mediate AIB uptake (17).

Incubation of HTC cells with 0.1 μM dexamethasone, a synthetic glucocorticoid, causes a dramatic decrease in the initial rates of influx of AIB. After a lag of approximately 30 min, the rate of uptake of AIB falls to approximately 50% of control within two hours, and to as little as 10% of control rate after 6-8 hrs incubation with the hormone. There is a concomitant fall in the capacity of the transport system (V_{max}) without change in the apparent affinity for substrate (Km). The efflux of AIB from HTC cells is not increased (17). Dexamethasone similarly inhibits the transport of alanine, glycine, and serine, which share the A-system with AIB; but has only a modest inhibitory effect on the transport of leucine, valine, tyrosine, or phenylalanine, amino acids which are transported primarily by the L or leucine-preferring system (18).

Dr. Roderick MacDonald in my laboratory has demonstrated that the steroid specificity for this inhibition appears to be the same as that for tyrosine aminotransferase induction in HTC cells (19). That is, dexamethasone and hydrocortisone are optimal inhibitors of amino acid transport; deoxycorticosterone is a suboptimal inhibitor, and 17α-methyltestosterone does not inhibit AIB uptake, but does block the inhibitory action of hydrocortisone or dexamethasone. Thus, it appears that transport inhibition is mediated by the same steroid receptor system involved in transaminase induction.

The inhibition of transport by dexamethasone is entirely reversed by removing the glucocorticoid, and partially reversed by antagonizing its action with 17α-methyltestosterone. The inhibition is also reversed by insulin. Insulin has only a slightly stimulatory effect on AIB uptake in untreated cells; but causes a three- to five-fold increase in transport in steroid-treated cells, which is maximal within two hours incubation with insulin. Like glucocorticoids, insulin appears to effect primarily the capacity of the transport system rather than the apparent affinity for its substrate (17).

Neither the effects of glucocorticoids nor of insulin appear to be direct ones on the membrane. Both the inhibition by glucocorticoids and the stimulation by insulin require concomitant protein synthesis, in that they are completely inhibited by the presence of cycloheximide which itself produces only a modest inhibition of AIB uptake (17).

It had been reported earlier by Ballard and Tomkins that dexamethasone increases the adhesiveness of HTC cells, by a process requiring both RNA and protein synthesis, and showing steroid specificity comparable to that for tyrosine aminotransferase induction (20). This observation, coupled with ours on the inhibition of amino acid transport, suggested to us that glucocorticoids might bring about a program of membrane changes analogous to reverse transformation. Therefore, we have also examined the effects of dexamethasone on the surface morphology of HTC cells. Glucocorticoids have been reported to cause an alteration in gross morphology and a decrease in the number of surface microvilli in RLC cells, a line of heteroploid cells derived from normal adult rat liver (21). In collaboration with Dr. Judith Berliner at the University of California, Los Angeles, we have demonstrated that, consistent with our hypothesis, dexamethasone decreases the number of microvilli on the surface of HTC cells in suspension culture, as assessed by scanning electron microscopy.

Finally, Weinstein and his collaborators have demonstrated that dexamethasone rapidly decreases the production of plasminogen activator by HTC cells (22). Plasminogen activator is a serine protease associated with the cell membrane (23), that is produced and released in large amounts by certain transformed cells. Glucocorticoids rapidly inhibit the production of the protease by process that appears to require concomitant protein and RNA synthesis (22).

Thus, it appears that glucocorticoids can evoke a program of membrane changes in HTC cells representing a phenotypic reversion of transformation, and including inhibition of amino acid transport, enhancement of intracellular adhesiveness, alteration in surface microstructure, and a decrease in protease (plasminogen activator) production. The HTC cell may provide a unique model system for studying the hormonal regulation of membrane phenotype as it applies to neoplasia. First, HTC cells are malignant cells which demonstrate several characteristics of transformed cells. Second, at least four of these phenotypic features are susceptible to hormonal regulation. Third, a great deal is already known about hormonal effects on these cells (15,24). Fourth, dexamethasone does not alter the overall rates of macromolecular synthesis (25) or growth (26) of HTC cells, so that one can study the effects of dexamethasone on membrane phenotype independent of changes in growth *per se*. This is in contrast to the situation in L-cells, in which dexamethasone also evokes a reversal of transformed phenotype (22), but inhibits growth and macromolecular synthesis as well (27). Fifth, HTC cells contain little, if any, adenyl cyclase or cyclic AMP (28), so that regulation of membrane structure and function operating by mechanisms other than cyclic AMP can be investigated. And sixth, it may be possible to isolate steroid-resistant variants of HTC cells. Thus, it should be possible, using both biochemical and genetic approaches, to study the hormonal modulation of those aspects of membrane structure and function associated with neoplasia.

ACKNOWLEDGMENTS

This work was supported by a grant from the National Institutes of Health (GM 15419). The author is the recipient of a Faculty Research Award (FRA-135) from the American Cancer Society.

REFERENCES

1. Pitot, H.C., Ann. Rev. Biochem. 35:335, 1966.

2. Pardee, A.B., L. Jimenez de Asua and E. Rozengurt, Cold Spring Harbor Conference on Cell Proliferation 1:547, 1974.

3. Imbar, M., H. Ben-Bassat and L. Sachs, Nature New Biol. 236: 3, 1972.

4. Burger, M.M., Fed. Proc. 32:99, 1973.

5. Emmelot, P., Europ. J. Cancer 9:319, 1973.

6. Patterson, M.K., Jr., J. Nat. Cancer Inst. 53:1493, 1974.

7. Pollack, R.E. and P.V.C. Hough, Ann. Rev. Med. 25:431, 1974.

8. Holley, R.W., Nature 258:487, 1975.

9. Beers, W.H., S. Strickland and E. Reich, Cell 6:387, 1975.

10. Fox, T.O., J.R. Sheppard and M.M. Burger, Proc. Natl. Acad. Sci. U.S.A. 68:244, 1971.

11. Johnson, G.S., R.M. Friedman and I. Pastan, Proc. Natl. Acad. Sci. U.S.A. 68:425, 1971.

12. Hsie, A.W. and T.T. Puck, Proc. Natl. Acad. Sci. U.S.A. 68: 358, 1971.

13. Hsie, A.W., C. Jones and T.T. Puck, Proc. Natl. Acad. Sci. U.S.A. 68:1648, 1971.

14. Gelehrter, T.D., J.R. Emanuel and C.J. Spencer, J. Biol. Chem. 247:6197, 1972.

15. Gelehrter, T.D., Metabolism 22:85, 1973.

16. Christensen, H.N., Biological Transport, W.A. Benjamin, Reading, 1975, p. 176.

17. Risser, W.L. and T.D. Gelehrter, J. Biol. Chem. 248:1248, 1973.

18. Gelehrter, T.D., W.L. Risser and S.B. Reichberg, In: Gerschenson, L.E. and E.B. Thompson (eds.), Gene Expression and Carcinogenesis in Cultured Liver, Academic Press, New York, 1975, p.190.

19. Samuels, H.H. and G.M. Tomkins, J. Mol. Biol. 52:57, 1970.

20. Ballard, P. and G.M. Tomkins, J. Cell Biol. 47:222, 1970.

21. Berliner, J.A., In: Gerschenson, L.E. and E.B. Thompson (eds.), Gene Expression and Carcinogenesis in Cultured Liver, Academic Press, New York, 1975, p.181.

22. Wigler, M., J.P. Ford and I.B. Weinstein, Cold Spring Harbor Conference on Cell Proliferation 2:849, 1975.

23. Quigley, J.P., J. Cell Biol. 67:347a, 1975.

24. Rousseau, G.G., J. Steroid Biochem. 6:75, 1975.

25. Gelehrter, T.D. and G.M. Tomkins, J. Mol. Biol. 29:59, 1967.

26. Tomkins, G.M., T.D. Gelehrter, T. Granner, D.W. Martin, H.H. Samuels and E.B. Thompson, Science 166:1474, 1969.

27. Lippman, M.E. and E.B. Thompson, J. Biol. Chem. 249:2433, 1974.

28. Granner, D., L.R. Chase, G.D. Aurbach and G.M. Tomkins, Science 162:1018, 1968.

ACTIVE FORMS AND BIODYNAMICS OF THE ANDROGEN-RECEPTOR IN VARIOUS TARGET TISSUES

Shutsung Liao, Stephen C. Hung, John L. Tymoczko, and Tehming Liang

Ben May Laboratory for Cancer Research
The University of Chicago, Chicago, Illinois

ABSTRACT

Studies during the last several years have indicated that androgen action in the rat ventral prostate is dependent on the formation of a specific 5α-dihydrotestosterone-receptor complex, while in some target tissues, testosterone rather than 5α-dihydrotestosterone appears to bind the functional receptors. In tissues with receptors that have similar affinities toward the two androgens, the relative availability and the differential metabolic activity of the androgenic steroids may be the major factors determining which form plays the predominant role in the androgenic responses. In some target cells, androgens other than testosterone or 5α-dihydrotestosterone may have their own specific receptors for their biological actions. The androgen insensitivity in various tissues of animals at old age or with testicular feminization and the insensitivity found in autonomous tumors, may be explained by low receptor content; in some cases, however, the qualitative and not the quantitative changes in the active forms of the androgen-receptor complexes may be responsible. Various androgens appear to bind to receptor proteins as if they are being "enveloped" by the latter. Such an interaction appears to cause the transformation of the receptor protein to the form that may be capable of functioning at the target site. There is no conclusive evidence, aside from the gross geometric structure, that any specific functional group or electronic structure is <u>absolutely</u> required for receptor binding and androgen action in the target cell.

Since it was first discovered that the ventral prostate of the rat can selectively retain 5α-dihydrotestosterone (DHT) in the target cell nuclei (1,2), and that this potent androgen can bind tightly to a specific cellular receptor in this tissue (3-7), considerable attention has been given to the receptor mechanism involved in androgen action in various target tissues.

Cellular proteins that can bind DHT or testosterone have been found in animal tissue such as the seminal vesicles (8-10), sebaceous and preputial gland (11-15), testis (16-18), epididymis (19-21), spermatozoa (22), and kidney (23-25). In addition, such proteins have been described in the submandibular gland (26,27), in hair follicles (28), and in specific areas of the brain including the hypothalamus, pituitary, preoptic area, and brain cortex (29-37). Other sites include the levator ani muscle (38,39), bone marrow (40,41), ovary (44), chick magnum (45), cock's comb and other head appendages (46), the pineal gland (47), and androgen-sensitive tumors (14, 48-50). Similar proteins are also found in the liver (51), lung, heart, and gizzard (46), where androgenic steroids may have limited effects. From these reports it seems clear that most tissues contain androgen receptors or receptor-like proteins, and that differences in tissue-specific androgen-binding activities are quantitative rather than being dependent upon the presence or absence of the receptor. One exception is the failure of many workers to find androgen receptor in muscle (other than the levator ani muscle), where androgens have myotropic or anabolic effects. Whether this is due to the technical difficulty of demonstrating the receptor or to the unique cellular mechanisms involved in the androgen action is not clear (cf. 94).

The original suggestion that DHT is the active androgen functioning in the rat ventral prostate does not necessarily imply that DHT is the only active natural androgen in various androgen-sensitive cells. In fact, there are now many indications that not all of the androgen actions can be attributed to DHT alone. As Attramadal et al (52) have reviewed, in some target cells, these differential effects appear to involve receptors that bind both testosterone and DHT, but the metabolic consequences and the relative affinities of the receptors toward the two androgenic androgens may determine their relative biological effectiveness. In tissues like the ventral prostate, seminal vesicles, and epididymis, the formation of DHT from testosterone occurs readily, whereas further transformation of the androgen to the 3α,17β-diol is a slow process. Therefore, DHT is accumulated and can bind to the receptor that has a low affinity for testosterone. In the kidney, uterus, ovary, submaxillary gland and certain areas of the brain, a moderate amount of DHT is formed, but is also rapidly transformed to the 3α,17β-diol. Since the receptors in these tissues bind both testosterone and DHT well, both androgens may be effective in these tissues. In the testis, the slow formation and the rapid metabolism of DHT as well as the receptor's preference for testosterone (as opposed to DHT) may make testosterone the major functioning form.

The androgen receptor in the cytosol of levator ani muscle was originally reported by Jung and Baulieu (38) to have a greater affinity for testosterone than for DHT, but more recent work by Krieg et al (39) showed that the reverse may be more likely. Since essentially no DHT is formed in muscle, testosterone may be the major receptor-bound androgen functioning in this tissue. The blood level of DHT can be as much as 20-30% of testosterone (53,54) but in some animals the blood DHT may be rendered inoperative by the serum sex-steroid-binding globulin that binds DHT more firmly than testosterone (cf. 3).

On the other hand, the biological action of certain androstenes or androstanes may involve different types of receptors. In the vagina, 3α-hydroxy- and 3-keto-androstanes stimulate the production of mucus by the superficial cells, while 3β-hydroxy steroids affect deeper layers and 3β, 17β-dihydroxyandrost-5-ene, and estrogens can cause keratinization of the epithelium (55). Shao et al (56) have found that some of these diols can bind to nuclear receptor-like proteins *in vivo* and in cell-free preparations. The same Δ^5-diol can also interfere with estradiol- and DHT-binding to the receptors in human myometrial and mammary cancer tissues (57). Receptor-like proteins that can bind 5β-DHT in bone marrow cells (41) or liver (58), and androstenedione in liver (59), have also been recently described. Evan and Pierrepoint (60) also reported that, in dog prostate, androgenic action may depend on a receptor for 3α,17α-dihydroxy-5α-androstane. There are also indications that the action of unsaturated androgenic steroids on certain brain functions may be performed by their aromatized products (estrogens) and by their binding to estrogen receptors (61). Recently, 3α,17β-dihydroxy-5α-androstane has been implicated by Walsh and Wilson (62) as having a role in the induction of benign prostate hyperplasia in dogs, suggesting the presence of a receptor for this androgen.

The above findings indicate that, in the same animal, androgen receptor proteins in different tissues have different steroid specificities toward testosterone, DHT, and other active steroids. Whether more than one species of gene is responsible for the synthesis of these receptors is not clear. If the synthesis of all androgen receptors is controlled by a single gene, some post-translational alteration of the protein or its association with other molecules may be responsible for the differences in specificities and affinities.

Other steroid-receptor proteins are known to be present in a wide variety of tissues (cf. 3). For example, glucocorticoid receptors are found in their classic target tissues, such as liver and thymus, as well as in those not normally considered to be target tissues, namely, placenta, heart and muscle. Estradiol receptor-like proteins have also been found in many tissues including the kidney, liver, rat ventral prostate (42,63,64), epididymis, and testis (64). The biological relationships among the multiple sets of steroid receptors in the same tissues or cells therefore deserve a more intense study.

The receptor content in rat ventral prostate glands decreases after the animals are castrated (6,14). This decrease is gradual (10,65) and follows the rate of regression of the prostate. Since the androgen receptor can be found for many weeks in castrated animals, the immediate action of DHT after it reaches a target cell may not depend on a specific androgen induction of the receptor protein. The androgen effect may be enhanced more rapidly, however, as the prostate cell grows, and as more receptor molecules become available to the cellular androgen.

Shain et al (66) have found in the rat that aging is associated with a reduction in the detectable androgen-receptor content of the ventral prostate. The receptor content in young mature rats (80-213 days old) had a mean value of about 11,000 sites per cell, but in the aged group (250-655 days old), the change in receptor content was not uniform and ranged from 14 to 90% of the values for the young animals. In old rats, the androgen-retaining ability of the cell nuclei and the tissues was low; this was believed to be due to the reduction in receptor content.

At puberty, the androgen-retaining ability of the hypophysis, but not that of the hypothalamus or cerebral cortex, increases (67). Testosterone and DHT can bind equally well to the cell nuclei of the hypophysis, but a decrease in testosterone and an increase in DHT-binding by the nuclei can be seen during maturation (33). The major nuclear-bound androgen in the hypothalamus and the cortex is testosterone, whereas DHT is the predominant androgen in the hypophysis. These findings are in agreement with the suggestion that DHT participates in gonadotropin regulation, but may not play a major role in hypothalamic sexual differentiation or in sexual behavior in some species of animals (68,69).

The liver has often been considered an androgen-insensitive tissue. Testosterone, however, has been shown to enhance the nuclear RNA-synthesizing activity of the hepatic cell nuclei of young rats (70). Castration of the adult male rat can also result in a gradual drop of the urinary output of hepatic $\alpha 2\mu$-globulin as well as of the DHT-binding activity of liver cytosol (50). Daily injection of adult castrates with DHT results in the induction of both activities. The androgen effects were not observed with immature and senile male or female rats, which cannot produce the globulin or the DHT-binding receptors. Estradiol administered to adult male rats results in complete inhibition of globulin synthesis and loss of the cytosol androgen-binding protein. It has been suggested that production of the receptor may be regulated in some way by its own ligands.

Rather extensive studies have been done on the relationship between androgen insensitivity and the androgen receptor content of the tissues normally sensitive to androgens. Since prostates or other androgen-dependent organs do not differentiate or develop in animals with testicular feminization (Tfm) (71-73), many comparative studies have been carried out with these and other androgen-responsive tissues. In male pseudohermaphroditic rats, the cell nuclei of the preputial gland (13), liver, and kidney (24) have a reduced capacity to concentrate radioactive androgen. The specific DHT- or testosterone-binding cytosol receptors are not found, or are present only in small quantities, in the skin fibroblasts from androgen-insensitive patients (74), in the Tfm-mouse kidney (5,75,76) and the Tfm-mouse liver (77). Others (26,78) have reported, however, that the cytosol of the submaxillary salivary gland of Tfm mice has a greater capacity to bind androgens than that from normal animals. According to Gehring and Tomkins (79), the kidney cytosol of Tfm mice which are deficient in high-affinity DHT-receptor has a large quantity of low-affinity and high-capacity androgen-binding components. They speculated that this may be related to the increased DHT-binding in the salivary glands described above.

Androgen-dependent mouse mammary carcinoma (Shionogi tumors) also contain androgen receptors. The content of the cytosol-receptor for testosterone was, in general, several times greater in androgen-dependent tumors than in some of the derived autonomous tumors (14,48). The lower cytosol-receptor content is apparently related to the poor retention of androgens in the nuclei of androgen-insensitive cells. Some of the insensitive tumor lines possess cytoplasmic receptors and show nuclear retention of androgen (50). Since some androgen-insensitive Tfm tissues and tumors appear to have high quantitites of androgen-receptor-like proteins, great care is needed in the use of quantitative data on the receptor contents as a guide to accurate prediction of hormonal dependency. Similar situations have been described for the estrogen receptor in mammary tissues and cancers (80,81), and also for the glucocorticoid receptor in lymphoma cell lines (82,83). In the latter, some of the steroid-resistant lymphoma cell lines had a normal ability to retain the receptor in nuclei, but the glucocorticoid-binding capacity of the cytoplasmic proteins was low or absent. In other insensitive cell lines, no qualitative or quantitative change in the receptor could be detected, but the receptor-binding ability of the nuclei was markedly reduced (79,84).

So far, biochemical studies on the molecular process of androgen action have been carried out largely with rat ventral prostate. While further investigations on this system may eventually provide the basic framework for the functioning of androgens in all types of responsive cells, the fine schemes that may be unique to and necessary for the specific androgen actions in varieties of target tissues may differ considerably.

In rat ventral prostate, the receptor appears to interact with the androgen as if the ligand were recognized from all sides and enveloped by the receptor protein. This is in distinct contrast to many steroid-metabolizing enzymes or blood steroid-binding proteins which generally recognize only a portion of the steroid molecule. Such a view is supported by structural considerations on the binding of many synthetic androgens with the prostate receptor protein (85-88); it also explains the very slow rates of association and dissociation of steroids from receptor proteins at low temperatures, as well as the very high affinity constant ($Ka: 10^{11} M^{-1}$).

An important finding in this regard is that 7α,17α-dimethyl-19-nortestosterone (DMNT) and 2-oxa-17α-methyl-17β-hydroxy-estra-4,9,11-triene-3-one are capable of binding to the androgen receptor more tightly than DHT; these androgens, like testosterone, have a Δ^4-3-keto structure in ring A of the steroid nucleus (85,86). Testosterone does not bind to the prostate receptor as tightly as DHT, apparently due to its bulkiness and lack of flatness, and not as the result of the Δ^4-bond <u>per se</u>. The 5α-reduction of this bond results in a flat molecule (DHT) that can fit better into the hydrophobic cavity of the binding site on the receptor protein. On the other hand, the removal of the angular methyl group at the C-10 position can make the androgen less bulky, and a further reduction of the Δ^4 bond becomes unnecessary for 19-nortestosterone derivatives to bind to the receptor.

In DMNT binding, the 7α-methyl group appears to play an important role, enhancing the binding affinity about four-fold (85). This may be due to the effect of the methyl group on the flatness of the steroid nucleus (cf. 89) or to the interaction of the methyl group with a specific binding site (M-site) of the receptor protein (85, 86,90). It has been suggested that a similar M-site may be present in the estrogen receptor, and that it may recognize the methyl terminal of diethylstilbestrol (90). The hypothetical M-site interaction strictly pertains to binding activity and not hormone action, since natural gonadal hormones do not have the methyl substitution.

A unique structural aspect of steroid hormones is that they contain an oxygen function at the C-3 position. Whether this group is <u>absolutely</u> required for androgen action is not clear, for many steroids without this oxygen group have been shown to be androgenically active (4). These steroids generally show very low binding affinity toward the prostate androgen receptor (84,89,92,93); this may explain their relatively low androgenicity compared to that of natural androgens. It is entirely possible that some of the 3-deoxy androgens are oxygenated and become androgenic. That 1,4-seco-2,3-bisnor-17β-hydroxy-5α-androstane (91), with ring A in an open form, is an active androgen indicates that oxygenation may not always be required.

It is possible, of course, that various 3-oxygenated androgens may have different affinities toward different receptors and may exhibit differing biological responses, as was discussed above.

With the exception of a possible involvement of 17α-hydroxylated androgens in the dog prostate (see above), the 17β-hydroxy group appears to be essential for high-affinity binding to the receptor and for androgen action (4,85). It is not clear, however, whether the 17β-hydroxy group is needed only for the formation of a tight androgen-receptor complex, or for the triggering process itself. For example, one can envision that the triggering action at a functional site involves a specific interaction of a cellular molecule with the hydroxy group of the steroid still bound to the receptor protein. This could weaken the androgen-receptor interaction and result in a structural reorientation of the complex. Whether the 17β-hydroxy group is required for the triggering action may be tested by the use of 7α-methyl-19-nor-17-deoxytestosterone. The methyl group in this compound could provide the necessary binding affinity, and perhaps the presence of the 17β-hydroxy group is not required for the receptor binding or the biological response. In this regard it should be noted that in the uterus estrone (which has no 17β-hydroxy group) binds at high concentrations to the estrogen receptor and is retained by cell nuclei, and presumably functions without being metabolized to 17β-estradiol (95-97).

ACKNOWLEDGMENT

The research in Dr. Liao's laboratory was supported by grants from the U.S. National Institutes of Health and the American Cancer Society, Inc. S.C. Hung was supported by a National Research Service Award from the National Cancer Institute, U.S. NIH.

REFERENCES

1. Anderson, K.M. and S. Liao, Nature 219:277, 1968.

2. Bruchovsky, N. and J.D. Wilson, J. Biol. Chem. 243:2012, 1968.

3. Fang, S., K.M. Anderson and S. Liao, J. Biol. Chem. 244: 6584, 1969.

4. Liao, S. and S. Fang, Vit. Horm. 27:17, 1969.

5. Mainwaring, W.I.P., J. Endocrinol. 44:323, 1969.

6. Baulieu, E.-E. and L. Jung, Biochem. Biophys. Res. Commun. 38:599, 1970.

7. Unhjem, O., K.J. Tveter and A. Aakvaag, Acta Endocrinol. (Kbh.), 62:153, 1969.

8. Tveter, K.J. and O. Unhjem, Endocrinology 84:963, 1969.

9. Stern, J.M. and A.J. Eisenfeld, Science 166:233, 1969.

10. Liao, S., J.L. Tymoczko, T. Liang, K.M. Anderson and S. Fang, Avances in the Biosciences 7:155, 1971.

11. Adachi, K. and M. Kano, Steroids 19:567, 1972.

12. Eppenberger, U. and S.L. Hsia, J. Biol. Chem. 247:5463, 1972.

13. Bullock, L. and C.W. Bardin, J. Clin. Endocrinol. Metab. 31: 113, 1970.

14. Mainwaring, W.I.P. and F.R. Mangan, J. Endocrinol. 59:121, 1973.

15. Takayasu, S. and K. Adachi, Endocrinology 96:525, 1975.

16. Hansson, V., O. Trygstad, F.S. French, W.S. McLean, A.A. Smith, D.J. Tindall, S.C. Weddington, P. Petrusz, S.N. Nayfeh and E.M. Ritzén, Nature 250:387, 1974.

17. Galena, H.J., A.K. Pillai and C. Terner, J. Endocrinol. 63: 223, 1974.

18. Steggles, A.W., T.C. Spelsberg, S.R. Glasser and B.W. O'Malley, Proc. Natl. Acad. Sci., U.S.A. 68:1479, 1971.

19. Hansson, V. and O. Djøseland, Acta Endocrinol. 71:614, 1972.

20. Tindall, D.J., F.S. French and S.N. Nayfeh, Biochem. Biophys. Res. Commun. 49:1391, 1973.

21. Blaquier, J.A. and R.S. Calandra, Endocrinology 93:51, 1973.

22. Wester, R.C. and R.H. Foote, Proc. Soc. Exp. Biol. Med. 141: 26, 1972.

23. Gehring, U., G.M. Tompkins and S. Ohno, Nature New Biol. 232: 106, 1971.

24. Ritzén, E.M., S.N. Nayfeh, F.S. French and P.A. Aronin, Endocrinology 91:116, 1972.

25. Bardin, W., L.P. Bullock and I. Mowszowicz, Meth. Enzymol. 39 Part D:454, 1975.

26. Dunn, J.F., J.L. Goldstein and J.D. Wilson, J. Biol. Chem. 248:7819, 1973.

27. Verhoeven, G. and J.D. Wilson, Endocrinology, 1976, In Press.

28. Fazekas, A.G. and T. Sandor, Fourth Intl. Congr. Endocr. Excerpta Medica, Amsterdam, 1972, (Abstract), p. 80.

29. Jouan, P., S. Samperez, M.L. Thieulant and L. Mercier, J. Steroid Biochem. 2:223, 1971.

30. Jouan, P., S. Samperez and M.L. Thieulant, J. Steroid Biochem. 4:65, 1973.

31. Kato, J. and T. Onouchi, Endocr. Japon. 20:429, 1973.

32. Kato, J., J. Steroid Biochem. 6:979, 1975.

33. Loras, B., A. Genot, M. Monbon, F. Beucher, J.P. Reboud and J. Bertrand, J. Steroid Biochem. 5:425, 1974.

34. Naess, O., V. Hansson, O. Djøseland and A. Attramadal, Endocrinology 97:1355, 1975.

35. Fox, T.O., Proc. Natl. Acad. Sci., U.S.A. 72:4303, 1975.

36. Sar, M. and W.E. Stumpf, Endocrinology 92:251, 1973.

37. Sar, M. and W.E. Stumpf, Science 179:389, 1973.

38. Jung, I. and E.-E. Baulieu, Nature New Biol. 237:24, 1972.

39. Krieg, M., Szalay, R. and K.D. Voigt, J. Steroid Biochem. 5: 453, 1974.

40. Valladares, L. and J. Mingnell, Steroids 25:13, 1975.

41. Mingnell, J. and L. Valladares, J. Steroid Biochem. 5:649, 1974.

42. Jungblut, P.W., S.F. Hughes, L. Gorlich, U. Gowers and R.K. Wagner, Hoppe-Seyler's Z. Physiol. Chem. 352:1603, 1971.

43. Giannopoulos, G., J. Biol. Chem. 248:1004, 1973.

44. Louvet, J.P., S.M. Harman, J.R. Schreiber and G.T. Ross, Endocrinology 97:368, 1975.

45. Palmiter, R.D., G.H. Catlin and R.F. Cox, Cell Differentiation 2:163, 1973.

46. Dubé, J.Y. and R.R. Tremblay, Endocrinology 95:1105, 1974.

47. Cardinali, D.P., C.A. Nagle and J.M. Rosner, Life Sci. 16: 93, 1975.

48. Bruchovsky, N. and Meakin, J.W. (1973) Cancer Res. 33: 1689, 1973.

49. Norris, J.S., J. Gorski and P.O. Kohler, Nature 248:242, 1974.

50. Bruchovsky, N., D.J.A. Sutherland, J.W. Meakin and T. Minesita, Biochim. Biophys. Acta 381:61, 1975.

51. Roy, A.K., B.S. Milin and D.M. McMinn, Biochim. Biophys. Acta 354:213, 1974.

52. Attramadal, A., S.C. Weddington, O. Nass, O. Djøseland and V. Hansson, In: Prostate Hyperplasia and Neoplasia, Alan Liss Publisher, New York, 1975.

53. Ito, T. and R. Horton, J. Clin. Endocrinol. Metab. 31:362, 1970.

54. Tremblay, R.R., I.Z. Beitins, A. Kowarski and C.J. Migeon, Steroids 16:29, 1970.

55. Huggins, C., E.V. Jensen and A.S. Cleveland, J. Exptl. Med. 100:225, 1954.

56. Shao, T.-C., E. Castañeda, R.L. Rosenfield and S. Liao, J. Biol. Chem. 250:3095, 1975.

57. Poortman, J., J.A.C. Prenen, F. Schwarz and J.H.H. Thijssen, J. Clin. Endocrinol. Metab. 40:373, 1975.

58. Lane, S.E., A.S. Gidari and R.D. Levere, J. Biol. Chem. 250: 8209, 1975.

59. Gustafsson, J.A., Personal Communication, 1976.

60. Evans, C.R. and C.G. Pierrepoint, J. Endocrinol. 64:539, 1975.

61. Naftolin, F. and K.J. Ryan, J. Steroid Biochem. 6:993, 1975.

62. Walsh, P.C. and J.D. Wilson, In Press, 1975.

63. Armstrong, E.G. and N. Bashirelahi, Biochem. Biophys. Res. Commun. 61:578, 1974.

64. Van Beurden-Lamers, W.M.O., A.O. Brinkmann, E. Mulder and H.J. Van der Molen, Biochem. J. 140:492, 1974.

65. Sullivan, J.N. and C.A. Strott, J. Biol. Chem. 218:3202, 1973.

66. Shain, S.A., K.W. Boesel and L.R. Axelrod, Arch. Biochem. Biophys. 167:247, 1975.

67. Monbon, M., B. Loras, J. Reboud and J. Bertrand, J. Steroid Biochem. 5:417, 1974.

68. Feder, H.H., J. Endocrinol. 51:241, 1971.

69. Swerdloff, R.S., P.C. Walsh and W.D. Odell, Steroids 20: 13, 1972.

70. Tata, J.R., Progr. Nucleic Acid Res. 5:191, 1966.

71. Perez-Palacio, G. and K.B. Jaffe, Pediatric Clinics of North America 19:653, 1972.

72. Meyer, W.J., B.R. Migeon and C.J. Migeon, Proc. Natl. Acad. Sci., U.S.A. 72:1469, 1975.

73. Bardin, C.W., L.P. Bullock, R.J. Sherins, I. Mowszowicz and W.R. Blackburn, Rec. Progr. Hormone Res. 29:65, 1973.

74. Keenan, B.S., W.J. Meyer, III, A.J. Jadjian, H.W. Jones and C.J. Migeon, J. Clin. Endocrinol. Metab. 38:1145, 1974.

75. Gehring, U., B. Mohit and G.M. Tomkins, Proc. Natl. Acad. Sci., U.S.A. 69:3124, 1972.

76. Attardi, B. and S. Ohno, Cell 2:205, 1974.

77. Milin, B. and A.K. Roy, Nature New Biol. 242:248, 1973.

78. Wilson, J.D. and J.L. Goldstein, J. Biol. Chem. 247:7342, 1972.

79. Gehring, U. and G.M. Tomkins, Cell 3:59, 1974.

80. Jensen, E.V., S. Mohla, T.A. Gorell and E.R. DeSombre, Vit. Horm. 32:89, 1974.

81. Jensen, E.V. and E.R. DeSombre, In: Advances in Clinical Chemistry, Academic Press, New York, 1976.

82. Lippman, M.E., S. Perry and E.B. Thompson, Cancer Res. 34: 1572, 1974.

83. Gehring, U., G.M. Tomkins and S. Ohno, Nature New Biol. 232: 106, 1971.

84. Sibley, C. and G.M. Tomkins, Cell 2:221, 1974.

85. Liao, S., T. Liang, S. Fang, E. Castañeda and T.-C. Liao, J. Biol. Chem. 248:6154, 1973.

86. Liao, S., T. Liang and J.L. Tymoczko, J. Steroid Biochem. 3:401, 1972.

87. Liao, S., Int. Rev. Cytology 41:87, 1975.

88. Castañeda, E. and S. Liao, J. Biol. Chem. 250:883, 1975.

89. Daux, W.L. and D.A. Norton (eds.), Atlas of Steroid Structure, Plenum Press, New York, 1975.

90. Liao, S., In: Rickenberg, H.V. (ed.), Biochemistry of Hormones, MTP International Review of Science, Biochemistry Ser. 1, Vol. 8, Butterworths, London, 1974, p.154.

91. Wolff, M.E. and G. Zanati, Experientia 26:1115, 1970.

92. Skinner, R.W.S., P.V. Pozderac, R.E. Counsell and P.A. Weinhold, Steroids 25:189, 1975.

93. Jung, I., C. Mercier-Bodard, P. Robel and E.-E. Baulieu, In: Goland, M. (ed.), Normal and Abnormal Growth of the Prostate, C.C. Thomas, Illinois, 1975, p.600.

94. Powers, M.L. and J.R. Florini, Endocrinology 97:1043, 1975.

95. Ruh, T.S., B.S. Katzenellenbogen, J.A. Katzenellenbogen and J. Gorski, Endocrinology 92:125, 1973.

96. Geynet, C., C. Millet, H. Truong and E.-E. Baulieu, C.R. Acad. Sci. D (Paris) 275:1551, 1972.

97. Siiteri, P.K., B.E. Schwarz, I. Moriyama, R. Ashby, D. Linkie and P.C. MacDonald, Adv. Exp. Med. Biol. 36: 97, 1973.

THE RELEVANCE OF STUDIES ON ANDROGEN ACTION TO PROSTATIC CANCER

W. Ian P. Mainwaring

Androgen Physiology Department
Imperial Cancer Research Fund
Lincoln's Inn Fields
London WC2A 3PX, U.K.

The classical studies of Huggins and Hodges (1) in which they reported the palliation of metastasing prostatic carcinoma by estrogens heralded a new era in the hormonal management of neoplastic disorders. This innovative work led directly to advances in the treatment of breast cancer and, to a lesser extent, in the arrest of malignant diseases of the adrenal and thyroid. Of similar importance in the historical context was the later work of Jensen and Jacobsen (2) on the specificity of the uptake and retention of tritiated estradiol-17β in rat uterus which, together with the advent of radioactive precursors for macromolecular syntheses, initiated a more penetrating and enterprising investigation of the mechanism of action of steroid hormones. Striking progress has been made in describing the selective binding processes or receptor systems for steroids and the mechanisms through which hormonal regulation may be expressed at a molecular level (3). It is propitious to appraise critically the impact and relevance of these experimental studies on the clinical management of prostatic carcinoma, particularly in the present economic climate where resources and finances are at a premium.

It is now generally agreed that the administration of estrogens suppresses the release of LH by negative feedback on the pituitary-hypothalamic axis (4), thereby curtailing the secretion of testosterone and reducing the circulating concentrations of plasma androgens. Despite warnings on the risk of cardiovascular complications in women taking protracted doses of estrogens in oral contraceptives (5), the widespread prescription of excessive amounts of stilbestrol for prostatic carcinoma has continued unabated, even in the face of serious criticisms of the putative benefits of a high estrogen regimen (6,7). Reports that estrogen administration after prostatectomy statistically reduced survival rates compared to the effects of prostatectomy alone (8,9) have prompted the publication of editorials on the relative merits of high-dose estrogen therapy (10,11). Opinion is currently divided. The efficacy of estrogens, particularly stilbestrol, in suppressing the secretion of testosterone to an extent even surpassing orchidectomy (12) is now well established, whereas other potential agents are singularly less effective (13). This laudable success must be balanced against cardiovascular morbidity and mortality, suggesting that the most pressing objective in experimental research is to develop alternative antiandrogens with less deleterious side effects than stilbestrol.

THE RELEVANCE OF EXPERIMENTAL RESEARCH TO BENIGN PROSTATIC HYPERPLASIA AND PROSTATIC CARCINOMA

Taking England and Wales as typical representatives of an urbanized western culture, disorders of the prostate gland give rise to demanding social and clinical problems. As originally stressed by Moore (14), prostatic diseases probably arise from changes in the utilization of androgens during old age. With quite exceptional case reports to the contrary (15), aberrations of prostate growth remain a characteristic feature of senescence (16) reaching such proportions throughout western societies (17) that one man in every ten in England, for example, will undergo prostatectomy sometime in later life (18). In contrast to earlier surgical practice (19), opinion now tends to favor transurethral prostatectomy (20), with a more limited but potentially increasing use of cryosurgery (21), for the treatment of benign prostatic hyperplasia. Simply to restrict the present discussion within the terms of reference of appraising the impact of fundamental research on the management of prostatic neoplasms, suffice it to say that chemotherapy appears to have a limited part to play in the treatment of benign prostatic hyperplasia. To substantiate this viewpoint, one of the more important steroid-related antiandrogens, cyproterone acetate (6α-chloro-17α-acetoxy-1α, 2α-methylene-4,6-pregnadiene-3,20,dione), has been submitted to extensive clinical trial against benign prostatic hyperplasia. While prostate regression was recorded by two groups of investigators (22,23), this was contrary to the clinical findings in general (for example, 24). The remainder of this article is therefore centered on prostatic carcinoma. For a review of the current status of the etiology and treatment of benign prostatic hyperplasia, the informative article of Tveter (25) should be consulted.

THE EPIDEMIOLOGY OF PROSTATIC CARCINOMA

In all authoritative reference works on aging and oncology (for example, 26,27), the epidemiological features of prostatic carcinoma are clearly defined. Based on a wealth of research and medical observation spanning over half a century, the four characteristics of this neoplasm are: a) a unique dependence on testicular secretions; b) a very dramatically higher incidence during senescence, ultimately representing the third most common cause of male mortality from malignant disease in all industrialized western societies; c) a dramatically lower incidence in far-eastern cultures or enclaves of yellow races in other geographic regions; and d) no clear correlation with occupation, wealth or social standing. In essence, prostatic carcinoma is an inexorable hazard of western maleness.

From the experimental standpoint, sufficient research is currently being directed only to the elucidation of the mechanism of action of androgens. Surprisingly, the influences of aging and ethnic origin on prostatic carcinoma have received deplorably little attention. In the present author's view, this is a serious oversight because it is unlikely that the onset of prostatic disorders is solely attributable to aberrations in the metabolism and utilization of androgens. Despite the fact that the life expectancy is now more assured world-wide through improvements in dietary, domestic and medical standards, aging research remains neglected. To a large extent, such aging research on the human prostate gland is limited by the lack of a suitable experimental model; this point is discussed in more detail later. Ethnic considerations should be pursued, however, as a matter of priority because they raise the critical issue of the acute sensitivity and specificity of androgenic responses. Extreme differences between races in the manifestation of androgen-sensitive processes are evident in the varying degrees of hirsutism, despite interracial similarities in the circulating androgen concentrations (28,29). While obvious limitations exist in the supply of prostatic tissue, worthwhile ethnic comparisons could be conducted on skin or hair follicles. The portents are favorable, because technology is now available for studying the binding of androgens in skin and sebaceous glands (30,31,32) and for culturing androgen-sensitive fibroblasts derived from human skin (33,34).

THE ETIOLOGY OF PROSTATIC CARCINOMA

Two areas of contention exist regarding the etiology of prostatic carcinoma and these are likely to dominate statistical and morphological discussions for some time to come. Predominantly based on the classical anatomy of the human prostate gland laid down by Lowsley (35), benign hyperplasia is believed to arise from the inner periurethral area whereas carcinoma originates in the outer lobes. Extension of this work by Moore (14) and others (36) led to the general premise that prostatic disorders originate in atrophic areas where androgenic stimulation was impaired. On the other hand, McNeal (37) has contested this concept, suggesting that there were serious limitation to the traditional model of the human prostate gland (35) and furthermore, that disorders in prostatic growth originated in foci of stimulated cells. This latter point has recently been corroborated by Tannenbaum (38). The question of androgen deprivation in senescence is discussed more fully in the next section. Over and above this moot point has emerged the extremely controversial postulate that there is a progression from benign prostatic hyperplasia to malignant carcinoma, as suggested recently by Armenian et al (39). If validated, the progression theory could completely alter our etiological conception of prostatic carcinoma and opposing views to such a causal relationship between hyperplasia and carcinoma have already been sounded (40,41). Evidence supporting progression, especially from an experimental standpoint, is extremely limited (42,43). Nevertheless, a higher frequency of nodular hyperplasia was reported at necropsy of carcinomatous prostates than in matched controls (44), and although a very indirect indication, urinary steroid catabolites are similar in patients with prostatic hyperplasia and carcinoma and contrast with those in healthy individuals free of prostatic disease (45). The importance of this etiological debate is illustrated by the recent editorial in the British Medical Journal (issue 5948, January 1, 1975). Such controversy is almost inevitable when important concepts are based largely on statistical evaluations and indeed the work of the principal opponents of the progression theory (41) has itself been questioned (46). This stimulating reassessment of the etiology of prostatic cancer indicates a healthy state of enquiry, but the matter should be unequivocally resolved otherwise the design of future research and the basic tenets of the cause of prostatic disorders will be placed in jeopardy. To complicate matters even further, the provocative idea that there is a familial or genetic predisposition to hormone-sensitive neoplasms also warrants prompt verification (47).

ANDROGEN SECRETION, TRANSPORT AND UPTAKE DURING SENESCENCE

In view of the correlation between prostatic disorders with both aging and androgens, considerable effort has been devoted to measurements of circulating androgen concentrations in senescence. Indeed, the development of specific and sensitive assays for steroid hormones, together with advances in our understanding of the transport of steroids in plasma (reviewed in 3,48) has been a major contribution of experimental research to contemporary clinical medicine.

Earlier ideas that reduced androgen secretion was a feature of male senescence (49) have not withstood subsequent evaluation by sophisticated analysis (for example, 50); on current evidence, the circulating levels of testosterone are essentially maintained even in advanced age. Based on earlier work by Daughaday (51), it is now clear that both testosterone and estradiol-17β are transported in human plasma by their high affinity binding to a common protein, sex steroid-binding β-globulin or SBG (52,53). From the effects of administering T_3 (54), together with studies on thyrotoxicosis and idiopathic hirsutism, it has been established that thyroid hormones regulate the synthesis of SBG and the levels of this important binding protein are fully maintained throughout life, even in extreme old age (55). There is additional evidence that the androgenic index or circulating free androgens, unbound to SBG, declines gradually with age (56). Taken overall, dramatic fluctuations in the secretion and transport of testosterone with age do not provide a plausible explanation for the onset of prostatic neoplasms. Furthermore, plasma levels of androgens have not as yet provided a definitive means for the diagnosis of these disorders.

Accepting this relatively unchanging androgenic milieu in male plasma, prostate disorders probably begin as the result of changes in the uptake, retention or utilization of androgens within the prostate gland itself. Save for consideration of the mechanism of action of progesterone in a limited number of species (3), androgen action is unique in that metabolism of testosterone to a diversity of products occurs within the androgen target cells. The human prostate gland is no exception to this general premise and is capable of forming abundant amounts of the putative "active" androgen, 5α-dihydrotestosterone (17β-hydroxy-5α-androstane-3-one) and other metabolites (for review, see 57). However, no distinctive deletion or error in testosterone metabolism can explain the prevalence of neoplasia in the human gland. A very significant milestone in the physiology of the human prostate gland was contributed by Siiteri and Wilson (58). In this penetrating study, they established that there was a marked accumulation of 5α-dihydrotestosterone in the prostate glands of men aged sixty years and above, whereas there was no relationship between age and the intraprostatic content of testosterone (58). Furthermore, the elevated concentration of 5α-dihydrotestosterone was particularly evident in the periurethral area where hyperplasia is initiated (58), either in the mucosal and submucosal glands of the prostatic urethra (36) or in the periurethral epithelium itself (59). This innovative work suggests that prostatic neoplasms may stem from a disorganization of androgen metabolism with age such that the prostate gland is under increased but localized androgenic stimulation. A higher concentration of androgens within the prostate gland relative to that in plasma corroborates this viewpoint (60).

This change of androgen concentration within the prostate gland with age could be attributed to either facilitated uptake or impaired release of testosterone, plus its metabolites, but neither of these processes have been unequivocally defined in any steroid-sensitive cell to date (see review, 3). The active transport of steroids out of cells has been reported (61,62) but it is believed not to involve further intracellular metabolism of steroids (63). Such exit processes have not been detected in the prostate gland but while testosterone must be converted to 5α-dihydrotestosterone to elicit maximum biological activity, by implication (63) the "active" androgen need not necessarily be metabolized further to terminate its action. Notwithstanding these speculations, it seems far more probable that the aged human prostate gland has a pronounced ability to concentrate androgens from the plasma. Until recently, the existence for an entry mechanism for steroids into cells was meager (64,65) but using the elegant superfusion technique, Giorgi and her collaborators (66,67) were able to demonstrate a specific carrier mechanism facilitating the entry of androgens into the prostate gland. Of outstanding importance was the increased ability to concentrate 5α-dihydrotestosterone in the hypertrophied gland compared with normal prostate (68). Similar findings were recently reported for a pituitary adenocarcinoma cell line in culture (69). Currently available evidence therefore favors the concept that prostatic disorders originate from androgenic stimulation rather than deprivation during senescence.

A MODEL FOR THE MECHANISM OF ACTION OF ANDROGENS

Based on experimental findings from the author's laboratory and elsewhere, a working model for androgen action is depicted in Fig 1; for the main part, the data were obtained from studies on rat ventral prostate gland. The salient features are as follows: a) Testosterone is transported as a complex with SBG (probably with corticosteroid-binding α_2-globulin or CBG in the rat and a few other species; for review, see 48), is released at the plasma membrane and enters target cells by a facilitated entry mechanism. b) Extensive metabolism of testosterone occurs to a diversity of 5α-reduced androgenic steroids. Of these, certain diols may regulate secretion but 5α-dihydrotestosterone is essentially bound with a high affinity to a cytoplasmic androgen receptor protein. c) Non-metabolized testosterone (or other metabolites) stimulates the intracellular synthesis of cAMP which in turn regulates an exceedingly restricted number of biochemical processes, principally those associated with the pentose phosphate shunt. d) Through a thermal activation step, the 5α-dihydrotestosterone∿receptor complex associates non-covalently with specific acceptor sites (DNA and its non-histone protein complement) within chromatin. e) The receptor complex triggers the expression of genetic information in a temporal sequence of integrated events, for

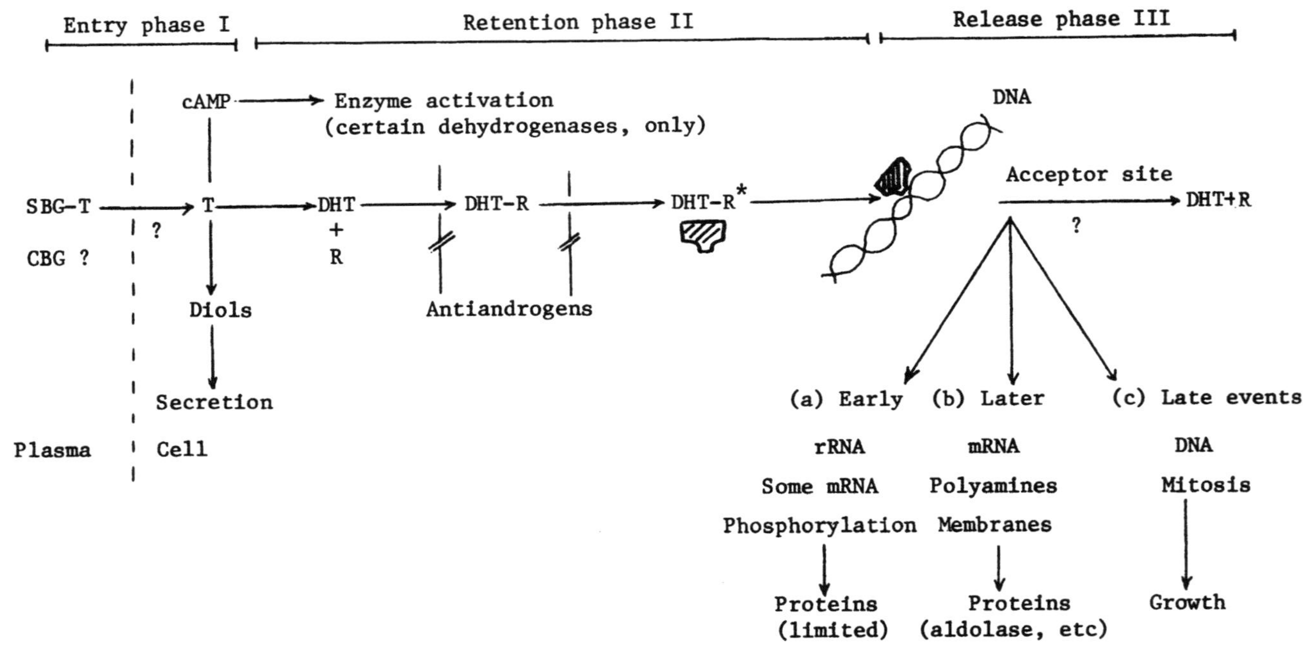

Fig 1. A Schematic Model for the Mechanism of Action of Androgens. T = testosterone; DHT = 5α-dihydrotestosterone; R = cytoplasmic androgen receptor protein; DHT-R* = activated receptor complex with a high binding affinity for the nuclear acceptor site; ? = reactions not fully understood. Particular emphasis is placed on the activation of genome, especially in terms of RNA transcription and DNA replication. As it stands, the model does not include androgen-mediated events proceeding by translational means or independent of the receptor system; furthermore, it does not explain the acute tissue-specificity of androgenic responses.

simplicity termed here early, late and later manifestations of the androgenic response. f) After considerable but nevertheless finite occupation of the chromatin acceptor sites, the receptor complex is degraded by a process which remains essentially unknown. g) Without exception, antiandrogens counter the formation of the androgen receptor complex and thereby negate all aspects of the hormonal response with but two exceptions; they do not impair androgen metabolism or processes modulated by cAMP.

EXPERIMENTAL ANIMAL MODELS FOR HUMAN PROSTATIC CARCINOMA

With the notable exception of the dog, carcinoma of the prostate is virtually unknown in other animals. This stricture has impeded the relevance and impact of experimental research because stringent species differences are biologically commonplace and experimental findings on other animals may be seriously misplaced in the context of human prostate diseases. A selection of the more important experimental models, with their limitations, is presented in Table 1. The dog prostate has long been advocated as a model system (70) and remains the object of widespread research today.

TABLE 1

Experimental Animal Models for Human Prostatic Carcinoma

System	Inducing agent	Limitations
1. Dog prostate (70)	None-spontaneous	Distinct pathologically from human neoplasms (71) Active androgen is 5α-androstane-3α,17α-diol, rather than 5α-dihydrotestosterone (72, 73)
2. Rat prostate (74, 75)	20-methylcholanthrene	Despite inducing a limited number of adenomas (75) the method is unreliable (77, 78)
3. Hamster prostate (79, 80)	SV_{40} virus	Not rigorously screened for prostate markers and despite some evidence to contrary (81, 82) a viral aetiology of human prostatic carcinoma is not unequivocally established
4. Rat (83)	None-spontaneous	Transplantable with metastases to lung; despite certain prostate markers being present, the androgen dependence remains to be clearly evaluated

Two serious limitations apply to this system; first, McNeal (71) has rightly pointed out that human and canine neoplasms are distinct in terms of origin, development and pathology, and second, Pierrepoint and his collaborators (72,73) now have irrefutable evidence that the active androgen in dog prostate is 5α-androstane-3α, 17α-diol rather than 5α-dihydrotestosterone. The carcinogen, 20-methylcholanthrene, has been widely studied as an inducer of prostatic carcinomas in the rat (74,75), but despite promoting histochemical and ultrastructural changes in the acinar epithelium (76) ranging from restricted hyperplasia to squamous carcinoma in certain instances, the induction was exceedingly variable and totally unsuccessful in other cases (77,78). The transformation of hamster prostate cells by SV_{40} virus has been reported to produce transplantable solid tumors on injection into hamsters of similar genetic karyotype (79,80). The tumors were not rigorously screened for biochemical prostatic markers and despite certain evidence to the contrary (81,82), the viral etiology of human prostatic carcinoma is not incontestably proven. It would appear that the best experimental model to date is the transplantable prostate adenocarcinoma reported by Pollard and Luckert (83). Three spontaneous, virus-free tumors have survived serial passage, with metastases to lymph nodes and lung; perhaps the only practical limitation to these tumors is their transplantation only into a Lobund variant of the Wistar rat. Successful adaptation to cell culture would be an asset and the androgen dependence of the tumor has yet to be clearly demonstrated.

MAINTENANCE OF THE HUMAN PROSTATE GLAND IN CULTURE

Because of the difficulties of obtaining a reliable experimental system, recourse will probably be made in the future to the development of cultures of human prostatic material. Interest in growing human prostate explants under defined conditions *in vitro* is by no means a modern day aspiration, for it was first tried by Burrows and his collaborators (84) over fifty years ago, with subsequent refinements suggested by Fell and Robinson (85) to suppress the outgrowth of fibroblasts. Outstanding success has been achieved in maintaining the prostate of the mouse (86) and rat (87) as organ cultures, to the extent that cellular differentiation, ultrastructure and secretion are maintained when the culture medium is supplemented with testosterone. These methods should now be applied to human material.

A brief summary of past achievements in culturing human prostate is given in Table 2, with the caveat that all the work has been conducted thus far on benign prostatic hyperplasia, whereas the long-term objective is to develop cultures of the less plentiful prostatic carcinoma. A cell line (MA 160) of prostatic origin has been developed (42) and maintained *in vitro* for over four years and forms solid, transplantable tumors in immuno-suppressed hamsters (88). On the evidence of the originators (42) and others (89), however, the tumor is exceedingly de-differentiated, lacking such prostatic markers as inducible acid phosphatase and the ability to concentrate Zn^{2+} ions selectively. The ability to maintain viable cultures of human prostate gland has been achieved by many independent research groups (90,91,92), with evidence of a satisfactorily maintained steroid metabolism (91), incorporation of thymidine (92) and several enzyme markers for screening hormonal responses (92). In all these cultures, however, the cells were not inhibited by antiandrogens (90) and did not respond significantly to exogenous androgens (91, 92). In other investigations (89) and particularly that of Webber (93), where detailed ultrastructural studies were performed, a diminution of androgen-sensitive markers, both enzymic (89) and morphological (93), was observed when the prostate cells were maintained in medium depleted in androgens. This appears heartening progress at first sight but regrettably the accelerated induction of acid phosphatase was not achieved when the cultures were supplemented with physiological concentrations of testosterone. At the present time, a stimulation of mitotic activity and acid phosphatase by androgens in cultured cells has only been achieved in one study, that of McRae and collaborators (94).

TABLE 2

The Maintenance of the Human Prostate Gland in Culture

Reference	Comments
Fraley et al (42)	Stable tumour line developed (MA-160), and gave solid tumours in transplantation into hamsters (88) Highly undifferentiated and lacking in prostate markers (42, 89)
Castro and Sellwood (90) McMahon et al (91) Harbitz et al (92)	Viable cells after protracted culture, with evidence of maintained steroid metabolism (91), mitotic activity (92) and enzyme markers (92). Refractory to exogenous androgens
Schroeder and Mackensen (89) Webber (93)	Well maintained cells on ultrastructural (93) and enzymic analysis (89). Prostate markers decreased in steroid-free medium but were not restored on addition of androgens
McRae et al (94)	Evidence for androgen responsiveness in terms of DNA synthesis and acid phosphatase activity

It is worth speculating how far the variation in androgen responsiveness given in Table 2 are the outcome of the conditions of culture, especially from the presence of exogenous polypeptide hormones. That the pituitary has an effect on the prostate gland beyond the influence of FSH and LH on the testis is well known and in certain species, prostatic atrophy proceeds more rapidly after hypophysectomy than castration (95). This pituitary influence is essentially mediated by prolactin (PRL), since this polypeptide hormone enhances Zn^{2+} ion uptake (96), citric acid accumulation (97), the uptake of testosterone (98,99) and may modulate testosterone metabolism (99,100). Also anti-PRL serum is purported to induce prostatic regression (101). Effects of insulin on the prostate are less clear but nevertheless enhance the viability of cultures by stimulating protein synthesis and other parameters (102,103).

Thus, although conditions have not been established for the reproducible maintenance of androgen-responsive human prostate cells in culture, significant progress has been made. If this may be achieved, such cultures would be the system of choice for screening anti-tumor drugs in the future.

ANDROGEN RECEPTORS IN THE HUMAN PROSTATE GLAND

As indicated earlier in Fig 1, the existence of a specific androgen receptor system is the linchpin of the currently favored mechanism of action of androgens. Extensive research has centered on the androgen receptors of benign prostatic hyperplasia and, to a lesser extent, prostatic carcinoma. A representative summary of this work is presented in Table 3. Two conspicuous points emerge from these studies. First, many authors commented on the heavy contamination of the specimens with SBG, necessitating the use of techniques for distinguishing between steroid bound to the plasma and receptor proteins; for example, electrophoresis (108), sucrose gradient centrifugation (106,107) and ammonium sulfate fractionation (105). Second, totally negative results were reported in two investigations (108,109). These failures are probably attributable to methodological difficulties; in particular, the tough hyperplastic nodules must be disrupted while preserving the labile receptor protein. Overall, high affinity receptors, specific for 5α-dihydrotestosterone are present in the cytoplasmic and nuclear compartments of the human prostate gland. The steroid specificity of the receptors was emphatically demonstrated by Mainwaring and Milroy (107) in a limited number of experiments conducted _in vivo_. In terms of physicochemical properties, the human prostate receptors bear a remarkable similarity to those reported in the male accessory sexual glands of experimental animals (for review, see 3).

In my personal and even iconoclastic opinion, it seems unlikely that measurements of androgen receptors will provide a practical tool

TABLE 3

The Identification of Androgen Receptors in Human Prostate

Reference	Tissue	Positive/Total	Method
Hansson et al (104)	Hyperplasia	Not given,100%?	Sephadex G-100
Geller and Worthman (105)	Hyperplasia	Not given,100%?	$(NH_2)SO_4$; Sephadex G-50
Rosen et al (106)	Hyperplasia	6/6	Sucrose gradients
Mainwaring and Milroy (107)	Hyperplasia Normal (non- adenomatous)	(14/27 (4/4 (	Sucrose gradients; Sephadex G-200
Steins et al (108)	Hyperplasia	None detected	Dextran-charcoal; agar gel
Mobbs et al (109)	Hyperplasia	None detected	Dextran-charcoal
Mobbs et al (110)	Carcinoma	Not given;100%?	Dextran-charcoal

in the diagnosis or prognosis of prostatic neoplasms. The situation contrasts sharply with that pertaining to breast cancer in women, where measurements of estrogen receptors have an acknowledged practical value in the management of the disease (111,112,113). My reservations stem from the following considerations. First, both the normal and neoplastic prostate gland contain significant amounts of receptors (107) so that quantitative distinctions of clinical value will be hard to draw. Second, the prostatic neoplasms appear to concentrate androgens actively (58,60,67,69) which, together with the heavy contamination with SBG (107,108,109), make the reproducible estimation of receptors a daunting task. Third, the removal of endogenous androgens and SBG is technically feasible but rendered difficult by the notorious lability of the androgen receptor proteins (3). Finally, the gross heterogeneity of surgical samples raises horrendous problems in terms of sampling and interpretation.

FUTURE CHEMOTHERAPY BASED ON ANTIANDROGENS

From the model presented in Fig 1, putative antiandrogens may counter the action of androgens at three points: a) testosterone entry; b) intracellular metabolism; or c) binding of metabolites to receptors. Gestonorone capronate is a candidate for suppressing the the entry of testosterone (114) whereas androst-4-ene-3-one-17βcarboxylic acid has been reported as a selective inhibitor of testosterone metabolism (115). Gestonorone may feature in clinical trials, but metabolic inhibitors are unlikely to be successful because the metabolic potential of the human prostate gland is such that inhibitors would be needed in extremely high intracellular concentrations. A comprehensive array of steroid-related antiandrogens has been developed which negate the formation of androgen receptor complexes to varying extents under conditions in vitro. As yet, none has the sufficiently high affinity for the receptor sites to have great clinical efficacy. This inconclusive outcome applies equally forcibly to the most enterprising steroid-related antiandrogen suggested to date, namely estracyt or estradiol-3-N-[bis(2-chlorethyl)carbonyl]-17β-phosphate, a subtle combination of an estrogen with a nitrogen mustard cytostatic agent. While this compound competed for androgen receptor sites under experimental conditions (116), it was not superior to estradiol-17β when tested clinically against advanced prostatic carcinoma (117) and similarly gave rise to cardiovascular episodes.

Non-steroidal antiandrogens may have a more promising future because they may satisfy the exacting criteria demanded in the clinical context, principally low toxicity, the absence of intrinsic hormonal activity, biological activity at low concentrations and ideally, no curtailment of libido. One such compound, N-(3,5-dimethyl-4-isoxazoylmethyl) phthalimide (118), has not been fully investigated even in experimental systems but flutamide or 4'-nitro-3'-trifluoromethylisobutyrlanilide, developed by Neri and his collaborators (119,120), is probably the most potent antiandrogen yet tested under experimental conditions (121,122). Results of its clinical evaluation are awaited with extreme interest.

CONCLUDING REMARKS

Remarkable progress has been made in extending our understanding of the physiology and molecular biology of androgens. Against this, many pressing aspects of human prostatic carcinoma remain essentially unsolved. Three areas of future experimental research appear to be of paramount importance: a) a deeper insight into the etiology and epidemiology of prostatic neoplasms in molecular terms; b) the development of more potent, non-steroidal antiandrogens; and c) the establishment of human prostate cell lines suitable for screening compounds of potential therapeutic importance.

Before the turn of last century, two enterprising surgeons advocated orchidectomy for the palliation of prostatic disorders (123,124) and another half century elapsed before a substantial improvement of their procedure was made (1). Hopefully, the widespread interest in cell biology and hormonal mechanisms will provide the foundations for further clinical improvements in the near future.

ACKNOWLEDGMENTS

I wish to express my gratitude to Mrs. Margaret Barker for her invaluable assistance in the preparation of this manuscript and to my colleagues, Dr. Richard Hallowes, M.B., B. Surg., and Mr. E.J.G. Milroy, F.R.C.S., for invaluable discussions.

REFERENCES

1. Huggins, C. and C.V. Hodges, Cancer Res. 1:293, 1941.

2. Jensen, E.V. and H.I. Jacobsen, Recent Progr. Hormone Res. 18:387, 1962.

3. King, R.J.B. and W.I.P. Mainwaring, Steroid-Cell Interactions, Butterworths, London, 1974.

4. Harns, G.W. and B.T. Donovan, The Pituitary Gland, Butterworths, London, 1966.

5. Medical Research Council Subcommittee Findings, Br. Med. J. 2:355, 1967.

6. Veterans Administration Cooperative Urological Research Group, Surg. Gynec. Obstet. 124:1011, 1967.

7. Byar, D.P., Cancer 32:1126, 1972.

8. Blackhard, C.E., R.P. Doe and G.T. Mellinger, Cancer 26:249, 1970.

9. Blackhard, C.E. and G.T. Mellinger, Postgrad. Med., March Issue, 1972, p.140.

10. Editorial, Br. Med. J. 8:520, 1974.

11. Editorial, N.Z. Med. J. 14:113, 1974.

12. Robinson, M.R.G. and B.S. Thomas, Br. Med. J. 2:355, 1971.

13. Robinson, M.R.G., R.J. Shearer and J.D. Ferguson, Br. J. Urol. 46:555, 1974.

14. Moore, R.A., J. Urol. 33:24, 1935.

15. Chiu, C.L. and D.L. Weber, J. Amer. Med. Assoc. 230:724, 1975.

16. Ashley, D.J.B., J. Pathol. Bacteriol. 90:217, 1965.

17. Doll, R., R. Payne and J. Waterhouse, Cancer Incidence in Five Continents, Springer-Verlag, Berlin, 1966.

18. Lytton, B., J.M. Emery and B.M. Harvard, J. Urol. 99:639, 1968.

19. Hospital Inpatient Enquiry 1970, London, Her Majesty's Stationary Office, 1972.

20. Argyrose, S., J.P. Blandy, J.G. Gow, M. Singh, G.C. Tressider and J. Vinnicombe, Br. Med. J. 3:511, 1974.

21. Elton, J. and B.M. Wright, Br. Med. J. 3:808, 1974.

22. Geller, J., A. Angrist, K. Nakao and H. Newman, J. Amer. Med. Assoc. 210:1421, 1969.

23. Scott, W.W. and J.C. Wade, J. Urol. 101:81, 1969.

24. Hald, T. and A. From, Scand. J. Urol. Nephrol. 6:157, 1972.

25. Tveter, K.J., Acta Path. Microbiol. Scand. Sect. A., Suppl. 248:167, 1974.

26. Cowdrey's Problems of Aging, A.I. Lansing (ed.), Third Edition, Springfield, C.C. Thomas & Co., 1952.

27. Raven, R.W., Cancer, Butterworths, London, 1957.

28. Kobayashi, T., J. Lobotsky and C.W. Lloyd, J. Clin. Endocrinol. Metab. 26:610, 1966.

29. Okamoto, M., C. Setaishi, Y. Horinch, K. Mashimo, K. Moriya and S. Ito, J. Clin. Endocrinol. Metab. 32:673, 1971.

30. Gomez, E.C. and S.L. Hsia, Biochemistry 7:24, 1968.

31. Eppenburger, U. and S.L. Hsia, J. Biol. Chem. 247:5463, 1973.

32. Adachi, K. and M. Kano, Steroids 20:567, 1972.

33. Mulay, S., R. Finkelberg, L. Pinsky and S.J. Solomon, J. Clin. Endocrinol. Metab. 34:133, 1972.

34. Keenan, B.S., W.J. Meyer, A.J. Hadjian and C.J. Migeon, Steroids 25:535, 1975.

35. Lowsley, O.M., Am. J. Surg. 8:526, 1930.

36. Franks, L.M., J. Pathol. Bact. 68:603, 1954.

37. McNeal, J.E., In: Pierrepoint, C.G. and K. Griffiths (eds.), Some Aspects of the Aetiology and Biochemistry of Prostatic Cancer, Alpha Press, Cardiff, 1970, p. 23.

38. Tannenbaum, M., Urology 4:758, 1974.

39. Armenian, H.K., A.M. Lilienfield, E.L. Diamond and I.D.J. Bross, Lancet 2:115, 1974.

40. Williams, R.D. and C.E. Blackhard, Lancet 2:1265, 1974.

41. Greenwald, P., V. Kirmss, A.K. Polan and V.S. Dick, J. Nat. Cancer Inst. 53:335, 1974.

42. Fraley, E.E., S. Ecker and M.M. Vincent, Science 170:340, 1970.

43. Sinha, A.A. and C.E. Blackhard, Urology 2:114, 1973.

44. Sommers, S.C., Cancer 10:345, 1957.

45. Marmorston, J., L.J. Lombardo, S.M. Myers, H. Gierson, H. Stern and C.E. Hopkins, J. Urol. 93:276, 1965.

46. Frei, J.V., J. Nat. Cancer Inst. 54:524, 1975.

47. Thiessen, E.U., Cancer 34:1102, 1974.

48. Westphal, U., Steroid-Protein Interactions, Springer-Verlag, Berlin, 1971.

49. Pincus, G., In: Engels, E.T. and G. Pincus (eds.), Hormones and the Aging Process, Academic Press, New York, 1956, p. 1.

50. Kent, J.R. and A.B. Acone, In: Vermeulen, A. and D. Exley (eds.), Androgens in Normal and Pathological Conditions, Excerpta Medica, Amsterdam, 1966, p. 31.

51. Daughaday, W.H., J. Clin. Invest. 37:511, 1958.

52. Murphy, B.E.P., Canad. J. Biochem. 46:299, 1968.

53. Steeno, O., W. Heyns, H. Van Baelen and P. de Moor, Ann. Endocr. 29:141, 1968.

54. Dray, F., I. Mowszowicz, M.J. Ledru, O. Crépy, G. Delzant and J. Sebaoun, Ann. Endocr. 30:223, 1969.

55. de Moor, P., O. Steeno, W. Heyns and H. Van Baelen, Ann. Endocr. 30:233, 1969.

56. Vermeulen, A., T. Stoica and L. Verdonck, J. Clin. Endocrinol. Metab. 33:759, 1971.

57. Ofner, P., Vit. Horm. 26:237, 1969.

58. Siiteri, P.K. and J.D. Wilson, J. Clin. Invest. 49:1737, 1970.

59. Mostofi, F.K., In: Campbell, M.F. and K.J. Harrison (eds.), Urology, W.B. Saunders & Co., Philadelphia, 1970, p. 1075.

60. Farnsworth, W.E., Invest. Urol. 8:367, 1971.

61. Gross, S.R., L. Aronow and W.B. Pratt, Biochem. Biophys. Res. Comm. 32:66, 1968.

62. Gross, S.R., L. Aronow and W.B. Pratt, J. Cell. Biol. 44:103, 1970.

63. Wira, C. and Munck, A., J. Steroid Biochem. 5:810, 1974.

64. Williams, D. and J. Gorski, Biochem. Biophys. Res. Comm. 45:258, 1971.

65. Milgrom, E., M. Atger and E.-E. Baulieu, Adv. Biosci. 7:235, 1971.

66. Giorgi, E.P., J.C. Stewart, J.K. Grant and I.M. Shirley, Biochem. J. 126:107, 1972.

67. Giorgi, E.P., I.M. Shirley, J.K. Grant and J.C. Stewart, Biochem. J. 132:465, 1973.

68. Giorgi, E.P., J.C. Stewart, J.K. Grant and R. Scott, Biochem. J. 123:41, 1971.

69. Harrison, R.W., S. Fairfield and D.N. Orth, Biochemistry 14:1304, 1975.

70. Zuckerman, S. and J.R. Groome, J. Pathol. Bact. 44:113, 1937.

71. McNeal, J.E., Workshop on Benign Prostatic Hypertrophy, N.I.H., In Press.

72. Harper, M.E., C.G. Pierrepoint, A.R. Fahmy and K. Griffiths, J. Endocrinol. 49:213, 1971.

73. Evans, C.R. and G.C. Pierrepoint, J. Endocrinol. 64:539, 1975.

74. Dunning, W.F., M.R. Curtis and A. Segaloff, Cancer Res. 6: 256, 1946.

75. Mirand, E.A. and W.J. Staubitz, Proc. Soc. Exp. Biol. Med. 93:451, 1956.

76. Aughey, E., R. Scott and I. McLaughlin, Br. J. Urol. 46: 561, 1974.

77. Brendler, H., Nat. Cancer Inst. Monogr. 12:343, 1963.

78. Chen, T.T. and C. Heidelberger, J. Nat. Cancer Inst. 42: 915, 1969.

79. Fraley, E.E. and S. Ecker, J. Urol. 106:95, 1971.

80. Paulson, D.F., E.E. Fraley, J.B. DeKernion and A.S. Robson, Endocrinology 91:396, 1972.

81. Cantifanto, Y.M., H.E. Kaufman and Z.S. Zam, J. Virol. 12: 1608, 1973.

82. Webber, M.M., O.G. Stonington and J. Lehman, Urology 1:561, 1973.

83. Pollard, M. and P.H. Luckert, J. Nat. Cancer Inst. 54:643, 1975.

84. Burrows, M.T., J.E. Burns and Y. Susuki, J. Urol. 1:3, 1917.

85. Fell, H.B. and R. Robinson, Biochem. J. 23:767, 1929.

86. Lasnitski, I., Nat. Cancer Inst. Monogr. 12:381, 1963.

87. Lasnitski, I., In: Pierrepoint, C.G. and K. Griffiths (eds.), Some Aspects of the Aetiology and Biochemistry of Prostatic Cancer, Alpha Press, Cardiff, 1970, p. 68.

88. Fraley, E.E. and D.F. Paulson, J. Urol. 101:735, 1969.

89. Schroeder, F.H. and S.J. Mackensen, Invest. Urol. 12:176, 1974.

90. Castro, J.E. and R.A. Sellwood, J. Path. Bact. 113:217, 1974.

91. McMahon, M.J., A.V.J. Butler and G.H. Thomas, Acta Endocrinol. (Copenh.) 77:784, 1974.

92. Harbitz, T.B., B. Falkanger and S. Sanger, Acta Path. Microbiol. Scand. Sect. A, Suppl. 248:89, 1974.

93. Webber, M.M., J. Ultrastruct. Res. 50:89, 1975.

94. McRae, C.V., R. Ghanadian, K. Fotherby and G.D. Chisholm, Br. J. Urol. 45:156, 1973.

95. Huggins, C. and P.S. Russell, Endocrinology 39:1, 1946.

96. Gunn, S.A., T.S. Gould and W.A.D. Anderson, J. Endocrinol. 32:205, 1965.

97. Grayhack, J.T. and J.M. Lebovitz, Invest. Urol. 5:87, 1967.

98. Lawrence, A.M. and R.L. Landau, Endocrinology 77:1119, 1965.

99. Farnsworth, W.E., In: Boyns, A.R. and K. Griffiths (eds.), Prolactin and Carcinogenesis, Alpha Press, Cardiff, 1972, p. 217.

100. Mawhinney, M.G., J.A. Belis, J.A. Thomas and J.W. Lloyd, J. Pharmacol. Exp. Ther. 192:242, 1975.

101. Asano, M., S. Kanzakim, E. Sekiguchi and T. Tasaka, J. Urol. 106:248, 1971.

102. Lostroh, A.J., Proc. Nat. Acad. Sci. U.S.A. 60:1312, 1968.

103. Fuller, D.J., K.M.B. Chan and G.H. Thomas, J. Endocrinol. 63:59P, 1974.

104. Hansson, V., K.J. Tveter, A. Attramadal and O. Torgerson, Acta Endocrinol. (Copenh.) 68:79, 1971.

105. Geller, J. and C. Worthman, Acta Endocrinol. (Copenh.) Suppl. 177:4, 1973

106. Rosen, V., I. Jung, E.-E. Baulieu and P. Robel, Compt. Rend. 248:4, 1975.

107. Mainwaring, W.I.P. and E.G.P. Milroy, J. Endocrinol. 57:371, 1973.

108. Steins, P., M. Kreig, H.J. Hollmann and K.D. Voigt, Acta Endocrinol. (Copenh.) 75:773, 1974.

109. Mobbs, B.G., I.E. Johnson and J.G. Connolly, J. Steroid Biochem. 6:453, 1975.

110. Mobbs, B.G., I.E. Johnson and J.G. Connolly, Urology 3: 105, 1974.

111. Wittlif, J.L., Seminars in Oncology 1:109, 1974.

112. Leclercq, G., J.C. Heusen, M.C. Deboel and W.H. Matteiem, Br. Med. J. 1:189, 1975.

113. McGuire, W.L., P.P. Carbone, M.E. Sears and G.C. Escher, In: McGuire, W.L., P.P. Carbone and E.P. Vollmer (eds.), Estrogen Receptors in Human Breast Cancer, Raven Fress, New York, 1975, p.110.

114. Orestano, F., J.E. Altwein, P. Knapstein and K. Bandhauer, J. Steroid Biochem. 6:845, 1975.

115. Voigt, K. and S.L. Hsia, Endocrinology 92:1216, 1973.

116. Hisaeter, P.A., Invest. Urol. 12:33, 1974.

117. Muntzing, J., S.K. Shukla, T.M. Chu, A. Mittelman and G.P. Murphy, Invest. Urol. 12:65, 1974.

118. Boris, A., J.W. Scott, L. de Martino and D.C. Cox, Acta Endocrinol. (Copenh.) 72:604, 1973.

119. Neri, R. and M. Monahan, Invest. Urol. 10:123, 1972.

120. Neri, R., K. Florance, P. Koziol and S. van Cleave, Endocrinology 9:427, 1972.

121. Mainwaring, W.I.P., F.R. Mangan, P.A. Feherty and M. Friefeld, Mol. Cell. Endocrinol. 1:113, 1974.

122. Varkarakis, M.J., R.Y. Kirdani, H. Yamanaka, G.P. Murphy and A.A. Sandberg, Invest. Urol. 12:275, 1975.

123. Rann, F., Kastrationens betydning i prostata hypertrofiens behandling, H. Aschehoug and Co., Kristiania, 1894.

124. White, J.W., Ann. Surg. 22:1, 1895.

SUMMARY OF CONFERENCE PLENARY SESSIONS

K.M.J. Menon

Department of Biological Chemistry
and Obstetrics and Gynecology
University of Michigan
Ann Arbor, Michigan

As an introduction to the discussion of steroid hormone action and cancer, Dr. Roy Hertz presented data derived from studies of experimental animals and humans on tumors that are induced by steroids as well as those secreting steroids, and those that are responsive to steroids. A variety of estrogen-induced tumors were described; high tumor strains of various species are found to be more susceptible to tumor induction by exogenous steroids than are low tumor strains. Dosage and duration of exposure also play a critical role in tumor induction by steroids. For example, there is a very critical period during organogenesis of the female genital tract for the induction of vaginal adenosis and possibly carcinoma. Steroid-producing tumors are restricted to those organs that normally synthesize steroids such as ovary, testis and adrenal. In the adrenal cortex the growth potential of the neoplastic as well as the normal adrenocortical cell is readily separable from its steroidogenic function. Hormone-responsive tumors provide examples of tumors that are responsive to endocrine therapy. Notable among these are the tumors of the breast and the endometrium which respond to hormonal treatment. A paradoxical case history of DES therapy of breast cancer was presented. Some breast cancers grow in response to estrogens, whereas others undergo regression with DES therapy.

Dr. Marvin Rich presented data supporting the thesis that breast cancer has a viral etiology. Mammary cancer can be induced by viruses in experimental animals and virus particles have been discovered in milk, human mammary epithelial cells and cell lines derived from human breast cancers. These viruses are type B oncornaviruses, whose genetic information is encoded in a 70S RNA and which possess reverse transcriptase and biophysical properties similar to those of other oncornaviruses known to induce neoplasia in several host species. In this regard, Dr. Rich added that the availability of a specific radioimmunoassay developed against a protein isolated from oncornaviruses would permit detection of viruses in body fluids and tissues in addition to milk and thus allow extension of these studies beyond non-lactating populations. The virus particles isolated from the milk of Parsi women in India, a group more susceptible to breast cancer than the Hindus, showed morphological properties identical to mouse mammary tumor virus (MuMTV). However, it has not been possible due to methodological problems to correlate the levels of oncornavirus in milk in populations with high risk of breast cancer, although several groups are searching in that direction. In attempts to develop in vitro systems for the isolation and propagation of human breast cancer viruses the development of a permanent cell line (MCF-7) from pleural effusion in a patient with malignant adenocarcinoma of the breast was described. MCF-7 cells were shown to synthesize a particle (734B) with all the characteristics of a known oncornavirus and DNA sequences were shown to be coded by the DNA genome of human cells and thus is a human endogenous virus. Further experiments in Dr. Rich's laboratory has demonstrated that the candidate human breast cancer virus, 734B, has some homology with mouse mammary tumor virus (MuMTV). Although in the mouse the tumorigenic potential of 734B is easily detected, it is not known whether the same is true in the human. The detection of specific association of such viruses or their antigens in human breast cancer may serve as a useful tool in its early detection.

Dr. William McGuire discussed the relationship between the presence of estrogen receptors in breast cancer and its responsiveness to endocrine therapy. Data obtained from several other centers around the world clearly indicate that the presence of estrogen receptor is correlated with the responsiveness of the tumor to endocrine therapy. Dr. McGuire made the important point that in some cases the metabolic lesion(s) may be at steps after binding of the hormone to the specific receptor, thus rendering an estrogen receptor-positive tumor non-responsive to endocrine therapy. Since estrogens are known to stimulate progesterone receptor synthesis, Dr. McGuire suggested that the identification of progesterone receptors in the tumor might be a more reliable indicator for selecting patients for endocrine therapy.

Dr. Merry Sherman discussed the analytical techniques which were applied in her laboratory for the fractionation and characterization of the multiple forms of steroid receptors in target tissues. Such techniques include analytical gel filtration, polyacrylamide gel electrophoresis, preparative ion exchange filtration, polyamine precipitation and sucrose density gradient centrifugation. These types of fractionation techniques are especially important because of the existence of multiple forms of steroid receptors in target cells.

Dr. Sherman applied these techniques to the characterization of estradiol receptors in breast cancer and elaborated on the importance of employing such rigorous criteria since slight contamination with serum might result in artifactual steroid binding in the cytosol. Her methods allow discrimination of serum and low affinity binding proteins from specific, high affinity, low capacity receptors in target tissues.

Dr. E. Brad Thompson presented data obtained from studies on human leukemic lymphoblasts. In his studies on glucocorticoid receptors in leukemic blasts, he reported that an encouraging correlation was found between the number of glucocorticoid receptors in leukemic blasts and the responsiveness of the donor patients to glucocorticoid therapy. It was recommended that the best test would be one containing some measure of receptor content with a measure of functional response, performed at the level of free steroid expected in therapy. Glucocorticoid receptors may provide a clue to the mechanism by which most leukemias escape from steroid responsiveness. Resistance to steroid therapy may result from multiplication of cells which lack steroid receptors or be due to selection of a receptorless cell population which already exists in the patient, or steroid or drug therapy may generate such a cell population.

Dr. Shutsung Liao delivered an overview of multiple forms of androgen receptors and the mechanisms of action of androgens. Although androgen action in the rat ventral prostate is dependent on its conversion to 5α-dihydrotestosterone (DHT) and the subsequent interaction of DHT with its receptor, in certain tissues testosterone, rather than 5α-dihydrotestosterone, binds to functional receptors. The relative availability and the differential metabolism of testosterone and dihydrotestosterone governs the predominant form that binds to the receptor in situations where both receptor populations are available for biological activity. As was proposed in the case of estrogen receptors and breast cancer, progesterone receptors and endometrial cancer, and glucocorticoid receptors and leukemia, it was suggested that androgen insensitivity in tissues might result from low levels or the absence of androgen receptors. In addition, qualitative changes in the active form of the receptor may be responsible for this insensitivity. No special structural requirements have been proven conclusively to be essential for receptor binding except for the gross geometric structure of the androgenic hormone.

Dr. Ian Mainwaring reviewed his efforts in uncovering the presence of specific androgen receptors in benign prostatic hyperplasia and prostatic carcinoma. Heavy contamination of the prostate cytosol by serum sex steroid binding globulin makes it necessary to apply techniques such as electrophoresis, sucrose density gradient centrifugation and salt fractionation to separate the specific androgen receptor from contaminating binding proteins. In addition, he cited two studies in which receptors were not detectable, probably because of methodological problems such as the toughness of the hyperplastic nodules to homogenization and the lability of the receptor. Dr. Mainwaring was pessimistic about the prognostic value of androgen receptor assays as a practical tool in prostatic neoplasms. This situation is quite different from the usefulness of receptor measurements in the prognosis of breast cancer, endometrial cancer and in leukemia. His conclusions were based on the fact that significant amounts of androgen receptors are found in adjacent normal and neoplastic tissue, rendering receptor determinations of questionable clinical value.

In the concluding presentation, Dr. Isidore Edelman reviewed his work on renal corticoid receptors with special reference to cytoplasmic and nuclear events. Three distinct high affinity corticosteroid binding proteins were described in the rat kidney. Type I sites selectively bind aldosterone, Type II sites specifically bind corticosterone and dexamethasone and Type III sites bind corticosterone selectively. The functions of these sites were analyzed in terms of a non-exclusive ligand binding, allosteric model. The predictions of this model were compared to the actions of agonists (e.g., aldosterone), antagonists (e.g., spironolactones) and partial agonists (e.g., 11-deoxycortisol) and to the effects of illicit occupancy. Based on the effects of DNA specific probes, such as actinomycin D, netropsin, ethidium bromide and proflavin sulfate, a structural basis of genomic acceptor activity was presented implying that the major groove of duplex DNA is directly involved in the attachment mechanism. The agonist activity is mediated by induction of specific RNA synthesis and antagonist activity involves inhibition of the induction process. These conclusions were based on the actions of aldosterone, spironolactones, cortisol and 17α-isoaldosterone in the toad bladder with particular reference to the effects on the synthesis of 9-12S poly A-rich RNA and on transepithelial Na^+ transport.

CONFERENCE COMMITTEE

David G. Anderson, M.D., Associate Professor of Obstetrics and Gynecology, The University of Michigan Medical School

Burton L. Baker, Ph.D., Professor of Anatomy, University of Michigan Medical School

Raymond E. Counsell, Ph.D., Professor of Medical Chemistry and Pharmacology, and Chairman of Programs in Medical Chemistry, University of Michigan Medical School

Thomas D. Gelehrter, M.D., Associate Professor of Human Genetics and Internal Medicine, University of Michigan Medical School

Raymond H. Kahn, Ph.D., Professor of Anatomy, University of Michigan Medical School

Robert P. Kelch, Ph.B., M.D., Associate Professor of Pediatrics and Communicable Diseases, University of Michigan Medical School

Merle Mason, Ph.D., Associate Professor of Biological Chemistry, University of Michigan Medical School

K.M.J. Menon, Ph.D., Associate Professor of Biological Chemistry and Obstetrics and Gynecology, University of Michigan Medical School

Scott E. Monroe, M.D., House Officer in Obstetrics and Gynecology, University of Michigan Medical School

George W. Morley, M.D., Professor of Obstetrics and Gynecology, University of Michigan Medical School

Mary F. O'Brien, M.A., Program Associate, Intramural Education, Department of Postgraduate Medicine and Health Professions Education, University of Michigan Medical School

Anita H. Payne, Ph.D., Associate Professor of Biological Chemistry and Obstetrics and Gynecology, University of Michigan Medical School

William B. Pratt, M.D., Associate Professor of Pharmacology, University of Michigan Medical School

Jerry R. Reel, Ph.D., Senior Research Scientist, Parke Davis and Company, Ann Arbor, Michigan

SUBJECT INDEX

Actinomycin D, 70,74-76

Adrenal Gland
- adrenalectomy, 29,31,32
- adenoma, 9
- carcinoma, 9,152
- corticoid secretion, 36
- cytolytic action of o,p'-DDD, 9
- hyperadrenocorticism, 9
- hyperplasia, 9
- steroid biosynthesis, 9
  - aminoglutethimide, 9
  - amphenone, 9
  - metyrapone, 9
- tumor regression, 9

Adrenocorticotropin (ACTH), 9
- pituitary, 9
- ectopic tumors, 9

Androgens
- action, 139-145,152-164
  - on gonadotropin secretion, 45,142,152
  - on hepatic α2μ-globulin, 142,143
  - on hypothalamic sexual differentiation, 142
  - on sexual behavior, 45,142
- anabolic effects, 140
- breast cancer therapy, 32
- comb-growth response, 3
- compounds
  - 5α-androstane-3α,17α-diol, 160
  - 5α-androstane-3α,17β-diol, 140
  - androstenedione, 120,141
  - androsterone, 41
  - dehydroepiandrosterone, 42
  - 5α-dihydrotestosterone, 37, 52,53,55,56,71,114,139-145,156-158,160,162
  - 5β-dihydrotestosterone, 141
  - 3α,17α-dihydroxy-5-androstane, 141, 160
  - 3α,17β-dihydroxy-5-androstane, 140,141
  - 3β,17β-dihydroxyandrost-5-ene, 141

Androgens continued -
- compounds continued-
  - etiocholanolone, 39,41,120
  - 7α,17α-dimethyl-19-nortestosterone, 144
  - 16α-hydroxyandrost-5-enes, 39,40
  - 7α-methyl-19-nor-17 deoxytestosterone, 145
  - 17α-methyltestosterone, 120,135
  - 19-nor-testosterone, 120,144
  - 2-oxa-17α-methyl-17β-hydroxy-estra-4,9,11-triene-3-one, 144
  - 1,4-seco-2,3-bisnor-17β-hydroxy-5α-androstane, 145
  - testosterone, 1,37,71,120,139-145,156-164
- effects on prostate, 139-145
  - benign hyperplasia, 141,153,154
  - carcinoma, 152-164
- insensitivity, 3,139,143
- metabolism, 37,39,40-43,45,141, 154-156,159,161
- myotrophic effects, 140
- preputial gland response, 3
- receptors, 3,139-145,157-160,162-164
  - affinities, 140,141,144
  - content, 139,142,143
  - specificities, 141
- SBG, 53,54,56-58,141,156,157,162, 163
- secretion, 36,156
- submaxillary gland response, 3
- testicular feminization, 3,139,143
- tissues containing binding proteins
  - brain cortex, 140,142
  - bone marrow, 140,141
  - comb, 140
  - epididymis, 140
  - gizzard, 140
  - hair follicles, 140
  - heart, 140
  - hypothalamus, 140,142
  - kidney, 140,143
  - levator ani, 140,141
  - liver, 140,141-143
  - magnum, 140

Androgens continued -
tissues containing binding proteins continued -
ovary, 140
preoptic area, 140
preputial glands, 140,143
pineal gland, 140
pituitary, 140,142
prostate, 139-145,157-160, 162-164
sebaceous glands, 140,154
seminal vesicles, 140
skin fibroblasts, 143,154
spermatozoa, 140
submandibular gland, 140
testes, 140
tumors, 140,143
uterotrophic action, 1

Anti-androgens, 153,161,164
androst-4-ene-3-one-17β-carboxylic acid, 164
estradiol-3-N-[bis(2-chorethyl) carboxyl]-17β-phosphate, 164
gestonorone capronate, 163
N-(3,5-dimethyl-4-isoazoylmethyl)phthalimide, 164
4'-nitro-3'-trifluoromethylisobutyrlanilide (flutamide), 164

Anti-corticoids
cortexolone, 120
progesterone, 120
spironolactones, 3,120

Anti-estrogens, 44,110-112

Avian Oviduct, 1
chick, 2,51,59-66,88,89
estrogen and progesterone effects, 2

Breast Cancer, 4,85,95,96-98,104, 152,163
Bittner's experiments, 17
cultured epithelial cells, 15, 21,22,24
growth potential, 22
MCF-7 line, 23-25
particle 734B, 23-25
pleural effusion, 23,31

Breast Cancer continued -
cultured epithelial cells continued -
ultrastructure, 21
death rates from, 16
DES treatment, 10,11,102,152
discriminants, 39
endocrine manipulation, 11,28-33, 39,85,152
estrogen receptors, 24,28-33,52-55,107,125,141,143,163
factors affecting incidence, 16
hormone dependence, 29,32,68
in experimental animals, 15
in mice, 17,23,24
malignant transformation, 28,29
membrane receptors, 29
NCI task force, 30,31,90
Parsi community in Bombay, 18,19
polymorphism, 15
populations at risk, 15,17-19
postmenopausal women, 30,39,43,53
premenopausal women, 43,52,54,56
progesterone receptors, 24,28,33
prognostic factors
menopausal status, 28,32
disease-free interval, 28,32
site of lesion, 28,30,32
protective effects of
pregnancy, 99
oral contraceptives, 99
Shionogi tumors, 143
steroid metabolism, 36-43
tumor regression, 10,11, 28-33,39

Carcinogens
latent period, 7
20-methylcholanthrene, 159,160

Cell Membranes
antigenic nature, 133
chemical composition, 133,134
density-dependent inhibition of growth, 133,134
glucocorticoid effects, 134
amino acid transport, 134,135
in cell division, 133
in malignant transformation, 133, 134
morphology, 133,134,136
phenotype, 133,134

Cell Membranes continued -
  transmitter and transducer, 133
  transport, 133,134

Cervix
  carcinoma, 5,99,100
  progesterone effects, 8
  squamous metaplasia, 8

Corticoids
  adrenal biosynthesis, 9
  breast cancer therapy, 32
  cellular actions, 114-128,134-136
  competition, 33,120
  compounds
    aldosterone, 120
    chlormadione acetate, 97
    corticosterone, 120
    cortisol, 33,37,57,62,71,119,120,135
    cortisone, 37,120
    deoxycorticosterone, 1,120,135
    dexamethasone, 33,115,118-124,126,128,135,136
    5β-dihydrocortisol, 120
    2α-hydroxycortisol, 120
    megestrol acetate, 97
    prednisolone, 120
    prednisone, 120
    tetrahydrocortisol, 120
    triamcinolone, 120
  effects on
    cell membranes, 134-136
    hepatoma cells, 114,126,134-136
    leukemia, 116-128
  metabolism, 37,39-41
  receptors, 114-128,141-143
  secretion, 36

Cycloheximide, 70,73,75,135

Endometrial Cancer, 4,8,85-90,104
  hormone dependence, 68
  induction by estrogens, 7,8
  in vitro progestagen action, 88-90
  pre- and post-menopausal women, 90
  progestagen receptors, 88-90

Endometrial Cancer continued -
  progestagen therapy, 11,85-88,90
  progestin-binding capacity, 11,90
  remission, 85,90
  squamous metaplasia, 8

Estrogens
  antagonism by progesterone, 1
  compounds
    diethylstilbestrol (DES), 6,7,10,11,30,52-56,95,96,99-104,109,144,152,153
    epiestriol, 42
    17α-estradiol, 120
    17β-estradiol, 30,33,37,38,42-44,52-58,68-76,87,107-111,143,152,164
    estriol, 42-44
    estrone, 37,38,42,43,52,53,55,109,145
    ethinyl estradiol, 96,101
    2-hydroxyestrone, 42,44
    mestranol, 8,96
    2-methoxyestrone, 42
    polyestradiol phosphate, 87
    sulfate esters, 37-39,104
  effect on chick oviduct, 2
  imaging agents, 107-112
  induction of
    adrenal tumors, 4
    breast cancer, 4,44,96,98
    endometrial cancer, 4,7
    ovarian tumors, 4
    pituitary tumors, 4
    progesterone receptors, 68-76,88-90
    renal tumors, 4
    testicular tumors, 4
    vaginal adenosis, 5,100,101
    vaginal and cervical carcinoma, 4-6,99-101,104
  post-coital contraceptives, 101,102
  prostate carcinoma therapy, 152
  radioiodinated analogs, 107-112
  receptors, 24,28-33,44,52-55,68,90,109,111,116,125,141-145,152

Estrogens continued -
secretion and metabolism, 36-40,42-45
target tissues, 28, 109-111, 141-143
teratocarcinogenic effect, 6,101,102

Estrogen-Progestagen Combinations
endometrial carcinoma therapy, 87,88,90
hepatic adenoma, 8
oral contraceptives, 95-99, 103,104

Estrous and Menstrual Cycles, 68, 85,86,90
steroid receptor levels, 68,69, 88,89

Gonadotropins
chronic gonadotropin
ectopic tumors, 9
trophoblasts, 9
follicle stimulating hormone (FSH), 45,162
luteinizing hormone (LH), 152, 162
prolactin, 162

Gynaecomastia, 37

Hepatic Adenoma, 8
nodular hyperplasia, 8

Leukemia
glucocorticoid effects, 116-128
glucocorticoid receptors, 116-128

Lymphoid Cells, 115,120,126,143

Lymphosarcoma, 125,126

Oral Contraceptives, 95-99,103, 104,152

Ovary
ovariectomy, 29,31,32,69,70
secretion of steroid hormones, 36,38,69
tumors, 96,97,103

Pituitary
adenocarcinoma cell line, 157
hypophysectomy, 29,31,32,162
tumors, 49,96,98

Progestins and Progestagens
antagonism by estrogens, 1
compounds
anagestone, 104
chlormadione acetate, 97
cyproterone acetate, 1
ethynodiol diacetate, 97
17α-hydroxyprogesterone caproate, 87
lynestrenol, 97
medroxyprogesterone acetate, 104
megestrol acetate, 97
norethindrone, 97,103
norethynodrel, 97,103
19-nor-17α-hydroxyprogesterone caproate, 87,88
progesterone, 2,8,33,57,59-66, 68-83,85-90,114,115,120
R-5020, 33
spironolactones, 3
endometrial cancer therapy, 85-90
effect on chick oviduct, 2
in oral contraceptives, 95-99
<u>in vitro</u> action, 86-88
metabolism, 37
mode of action, 85-90
receptors, 24,28,33,51,59-66,68-83,88-90
association constant, 77-78,89
equilibrium dialysis, 77,78, 88-90
nuclear, 80-83,89
physicochemical properties, 59-66,68-83,89
purification, 89
regulation of synthesis, 68-76,88,89
stability, 77,78,89
steroid specificity, 71,89
structure, 59-66,76-80
secretion, 36

Prostate
androgen action, 139-145,152-164
androgen receptors, 139-145, 157-160,162-164
benign hyperplasia, 141,153, 155,160,162
chemotherapy, 153
carcinoma, 85,152-164
animal models, 159,160
anti-androgens, 153,163,164
DES therapy, 152,153
diagnosis and prognosis, 163
epidemiology, 154,164
etiology, 153-155,164
endocrine manipulation, 85,102, 162
prostatectomy, 153
senescence, 153-157
tissue and cell cultures, 160-162

Rat Hepatoma Cell Line (HTC), 114,126,134
adhesiveness, 135
enzyme induction, 114,134,135
glucocorticoid effects, 114, 126,134,135
insulin effects, 134,135
plasminogen activator, 136

Reverse Transformation, 134-136
inhibition by colcemid and cytochalasin B, 134

Steroid-Binding Proteins, 51
applications, 28-33,51,88-90, 116,122-128,162-164
characterization
ammonium sulfate fractionation, 89,162
charcoal-dextran assays, 52,55
density gradient centrifugation, 51,61,62,65,72,74, 76-83,162
Ferguson plot analysis, 58-60
gel electrophoresis, 51,55-62, 162
gel filtration, 51,52-55,64, 78,79,82,83

Steroid-Binding Proteins Continued -
ion exchange filtration, 51, 62-65
polyamine precipitation, 51, 64,65
intracellular
androgen receptors, 139-145, 157-160,162-164
estrogen receptors, 24,28-33, 52-55
progesterone receptors, 24,28, 33,59-66,68-83,88-90
multiple forms, 51,59-66, 76-80
serum, 51,52-59,144
albumin, 52-54,56-58
CBG, 57,62,118,157
SBG, 53,54,56-58,141,156,157, 162,163

Steroid Metabolism
adipose tissue, 37,42
adrenal, 36
breast cancer, 36-46
enzymes involved, 37,38,40,41,43, 44,46,144
excretion, 37
female and male patterns, 45
FSH effects, 45
hepatic, 37,38,42,45
metabolites, 36-46
ovarian, 36
plasma levels of steroids, 37
postmenopausal, 37,38,43
premenopausal, 37,38,43
radioimmunoassay, 44

Testis
castration, 142,153,162,164
tumors, 9,96

Tumors
experimentally-induced, 4
hormone-dependent, 28
ionizing radiation, 7,11
steroid-induced, 1,4,5
steroid-producing, 1,9
steroid-responsive, 1,11,28-33, 85-90
therapeutic manipulation, 9,11, 28-33,90

Tumors Continued -
tissue
adrenal, 4,9,152
bone marrow, 4
breast, 4,10,11,15-25,28-33, 96-98
bronchogenic, 9
gastro-intestinal, 9
hepatic, 8
mammary, 4,44,96
melanomas, 9
ovarian, 4,9,96,103
pituitary, 4,9,96-98
renal, 4
estrogen-induced, 4,11
testis, 9,96
thyroid, 152
trophoblastic, 9
uterus, 4,85-90,96,97,99,104

Turner's Syndrome, 7,8
XO and mosaic karyotypes, 8

Uterus
cancer, 85-90,96,97,99,104
hysterectomy, 88
species
guinea pig, 68,77-83,88,89
hamster, 68-76,88,89
human, 85-90,141
mouse, 68,88
rabbit, 1,77,78,80,88
rat, 68,88,89,107-112
sheep, 88
steroid receptors, 24,28-33,51-55,59-66,68-83,88-90,109, 111

Vagina
adenosis, 5,100,101
carcinoma, 4-6,100,101,104
DES
latent period, 7
teratocarcinogenic effect, 6, 101
estrogen action, 141
organogenesis, 5
Müllerian derivatives, 8
progesterone receptors, 68

Viruses
antigens, 17,20
Bittner's experiments, 17
breast cancer, 15,17,21-24
coat proteins, 20
cores, 20,21
density gradient centrifugation, 20
detection
biochemical, 19,22,23
immunological, 19-22,25
morphological, 19
endogenous, 17
genetic information, 17
in milk, 17,19-23
isolation and propagation, 23
leukemia, 23
mouse mammary tumor (MuMTV), 17-19,21,23,25
particles, 15,17-22
734B, 23,24
prostate, 159,160
reverse transcriptase, 17,19-21,23
synthesis, 21,23,24
transmission, 17
type B oncornaviruses, 17-20,23

MIX
Papier aus verantwortungsvollen Quellen
Paper from responsible sources
FSC® C105338
FSC
www.fsc.org

If you have any concerns about our products,
you can contact us on
ProductSafety@springernature.com

In case Publisher is established outside the EU,
the EU authorized representative is:
Springer Nature Customer Service Center GmbH
Europaplatz 3, 69115 Heidelberg, Germany

Printed by Libri Plureos GmbH
in Hamburg, Germany